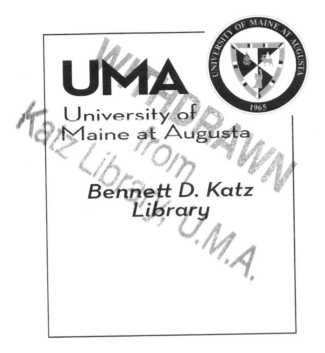

Black Dogs and Blue Words

Black Dogs and Blue Words

Depression and Gender in the Age of Self-Care

KIMBERLY K. EMMONS

RUTGERS UNIVERSITY PRESS

NEW BRUNSWICK, NEW JERSEY, AND LONDON

LIBRARY OF CONGRESS CATALOGING-IN-PUBLICATION DATA

Emmons, Kimberly, 1972–
    Black dogs and blue words : depression and gender in the age of self-care /
Kimberly K. Emmons.
        p. ; cm.
    Includes bibliographical references and index.
    ISBN 978–0–8135–4720–6 (hardcover : alk. paper)
    I. Depression in women.   2. Mental illness in mass media.   I. Title.
[DNLM: I. Depressive Disorder—psychology.   2. Advertising as Topic.
3. Communications Media.   4. Self Care.   5. Women—psychology.
    WM 171 E535b 2010]
    RC537.E46   2010
    616.85′270082—dc22   2009021737

A British Cataloging-in-Publication record for this book is
available from the British Library.

Visit our Web site: http://rutgerspress.rutgers.edu

Manufactured in the United States of America

To the memory of my father,
Steven L. Emmons

CONTENTS

ILLUSTRATIONS AND TABLES

ACKNOWLEDGMENTS

Writing is a solitary and a social endeavor: I owe a great debt to many who have offered me the invaluable gifts of time, support, and intellectual engagement. First among those whose voices have resonated throughout my writing process are the women who agreed to be interviewed and who shared their experiences and expertise with me. For their insights, humor, and careful articulations, I thank them. At the University of Washington, my teachers and colleagues nurtured my sometimes quirky love of language and supported my investigations with always the right touch of enthusiasm and critique. This project simply would not have been possible without Gail Stygall, Anis Bawarshi, Anne Curzan, and George Dillon. For moral support and the best skeptic's corner a writer could ask for, I am additionally indebted to my compatriots from Seattle, the Dames: Tamiko Nimura, Brandy Parris, and Brooke Stafford.

I am grateful to members of the Case Western Reserve faculty, among them many whom I am honored to call friends as well as colleagues. Special thanks to William Siebenschuh, who brought *le chat bleu* to my attention; to Todd Oakley, Athena Vrettos, and Martha Woodmansee, who each offered mentoring and camaraderie; to Christopher Flint, an office neighbor whose good humor was always appreciated (and whose patience for my questions never seemed to run out); and to Jonathan Sadowsky, for reading my work and for organizing the "Meanings of the Biomedical Mind" conference, which shaped my thinking about interdisciplinarity. For a dose of the walking cure, Thrity Umrigar's timing has always been impeccable; and for their general good humor, I thank each of my English colleagues. Above all, though, I thank Kurt Koenigsberger, whose friendship and editorial advice, in equal measures, guided this project from beginning to end. Without his support, humor, and willingness to read (and reread) portions of this project, it and I would have been lost.

Case Western Reserve has supported my research with several faculty development grants, and I am grateful to the W. P. Jones Fund and the Baker-Nord Center for the Humanities' Foreign Travel Grant program for supporting this project. Christine Mueri generously spent a semester working as my research assistant, and it is through her efforts and the generosity of Hara Estroff Marano that I was able to use the articles in *Blues Buster* in my analysis.

An earlier version of chapter 6 appeared in *The Rhetoric of Healthcare: Essays Toward a New Disciplinary Inquiry*, edited by Barbara Heifferon and Stuart C. Brown (Cresskill, N.J.: Hampton Press, 2008). I am grateful for the opportunity to revisit that material in this context. For her initial interest in this project, her writing advice, and her endless patience, I thank my editor at Rutgers University Press, Doreen Valentine. The readers of the first draft of this manuscript were also incredibly generous with their insights and time. In addition, I am particularly grateful to the CCCC Medical Rhetoric special interest group and to its fearless leader, Barbara Heifferon.

Finally, to the members of my family, each of whom has seen me less often and more anxious than any of us would have liked as a result of this project: thank you for believing in me. From the bottom of my heart, I thank Teri, Tom, Natalie, and Gabrielle Shultz, whose stories, pictures, and not infrequent visits have been a lifeline; Pam and Doug Smith, who offered encouragement and perspective when I could not muster them for myself; and the rest of my extended family. In addition to those who are genetically predisposed to love and support me, I am equally grateful to the friends who have been family to me: Shelagh and Mark Anson, Julia and Jay Crisfield, Michelle and Glen McGorty, Kristalee and Nils Overdahl, Sara and Brent Roberts, Brooke Stafford, and Margaret and David Wooll.

In the midst of writing this book, I have been triply fortunate. I am more grateful than they can know to William, Anna, and Magdalena Claspy for letting me into their family and for becoming a part of my own. I look forward with great excitement to the adventures we will have and the stories we will write together. To William, especially, whose love gives me hope that tomorrow will be even better than today: thank you, thank you, thank you.

Black Dogs and Blue Words

Introduction

Depression and Gender in the Age of Self-Care

As a "mental illness," depression sits at the intersection of physical, cognitive, and emotional realities; it is particularly vulnerable to the means of its own articulation. Without diagnostics such as blood tests or X-ray imaging, depression becomes visible or remains invisible through the language used to describe it. That language—from pharmaceutical advertising slogans to epidemiological models of the illness's frequency, from colloquial phrases such as "feeling the blues" to diagnostic terminology such as "psychomotor agitation or retardation"—both reflects and shapes contemporary attitudes toward health and illness, and in particular toward gendered expectations of who is vulnerable and of whose responsibility it is to maintain individual well-being. In the decade spanning the turn of the twenty-first century, public talk about depression seemed ubiquitous in the United States. Direct-to-consumer advertisements for antidepressant medications began to appear in print magazines and on the radio and television, as a result of a 1997 Food and Drug Administration (FDA) ruling that relaxed restrictions on this form of marketing. Peter Kramer's best-selling book *Listening to Prozac*, originally published in 1993, was re-released with a new afterword in 1997. And, Elizabeth Wurtzel's popular memoir, *Prozac Nation*, published in 1994, was made into a feature film starring Christina Ricci and Jason Biggs in 2001. Indeed, after the 1987 FDA approval of Prozac, the first of a new class of antidepressants, depression became a much more commonly discussed illness. In his 2001 memoir/encyclopedia of depression, Andrew Solomon remarks that "everyone and his uncle Bob seemed to be getting depressed and battling depression and *talking about battling depression.*"[1] This cacophony produced a sense of progress—depression was no longer a shameful secret—and it fostered a series of rhetorical forms that articulated the illness and the identities of its sufferers. Such language patterns, for example, the definitions, metaphors, stock characters, and diagnostic genres that recur throughout talk about the illness, constitute a discourse of depression that encourages what I call "self-doctoring"—an increased attention to one's own health and, indeed, one's gendered self.

Practices of self-doctoring define the contemporary mental health experience and shape its activities and interventions. In a 2007 *New Yorker* cartoon by William Haefeli, a woman seated at her computer is asked by the man who walks behind her, "How's the self-diagnosis coming?" (figure 1).[2] The vignette is funny because it so succinctly captures the migration of medical authority from doctor's office to individual, computer-mediated reflection. The woman's activity—described by her companion as "self-diagnosis"—can be read in at least two ways. She is serving as her own doctor, diagnosing her own potential illness and thereby acquiring the authority traditionally granted to medical professionals. And, she is also investigating her *self*, measuring it against a standard provided by the information she consumes online. In each case, though, texts—presumably

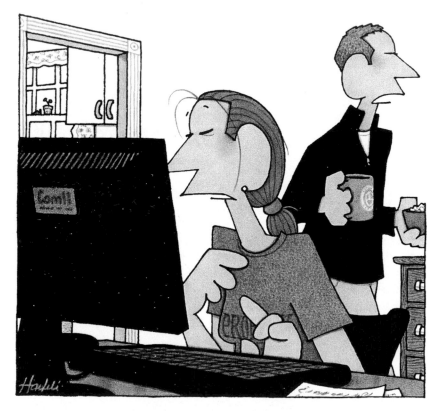

"How's the self-diagnosis coming?"

FIGURE 1. Self-diagnosis cartoon, 2007. (© The New Yorker Collection 2007 William Haefeli from cartoonbank.com. All Rights Reserved)

the self-diagnostic quizzes readily available on consumer Web sites—mediate her "expert" and "patient" identities. The cartoon displays a growing reliance on interactions between isolated individuals and the texts that construct health and illness. The woman's companion does not look at her as he passes; there is no indication that she is in dialogue with anyone else; her self-diagnosis is a monological practice (which is part of what the cartoon parodies).

The woman's apparent self-reliance reflects a growing sense of patient empowerment in the late twentieth century, particularly in the realm of mental health and illness. Recent advances in treatments for mental illnesses such as depression have been widely publicized and discussed in popular media, and information about both illnesses and treatments have become readily available to individual patients.

This self-reliance results in part from the rhetoric of patient self-empowerment that characterized the late twentieth century, particularly in the realm of mental health and illness. As health-care information has become more accessible, a new regime of self-doctoring practices has developed, one that Amy Harmon documents in the *New York Times* as a trend not only toward self-diagnosis but also toward self-*medication*. Harmon writes: "For a sizable group of people in their 20s and 30s, deciding on their own what drugs to take—in particular, stimulants, antidepressants and other psychiatric medications—is becoming the norm. Confident of their abilities and often skeptical of psychiatrists' expertise, they choose to rely on their own research and each other's experience in treating problems like depression, fatigue, anxiety or a lack of concentration. A medical degree, in their view, is useful, but not essential, and certainly not sufficient."[3] For these individuals, illnesses such as depression become research projects as well as, or perhaps more than, medical conditions, and this is one result of the availability of health-care information in forms accessible to nonspecialists. Harmon's young people want "to feel better—less depressed, less stressed out, more focused, better rested," and they fulfill these desires by self-doctoring practices that include monitoring individual symptoms, researching pharmaceuticals and illnesses, and using their personal experiences as diagnostic authority. Language underwrites these practices of self-doctoring; it provides the justification for attending to the self as a site for medical, often pharmaceutical, intervention.

Not unlike Harmon's subjects, we are all doctors, or at least dispensers of medical wisdom, in this new age of self-care. Whether we research potential ailments online, note particular pharmaceutical advertisements in favorite magazines or on television, or consult health-care encyclopedias and self-help texts, we are preoccupied not only with our potential self-diagnoses but also in sharing the results of our investigations. That we can now casually discuss prescriptions for Prozac and courses of hormone replacement therapy indicates, on one hand, a comfort and openness with both health and illness as parts of daily life and, on the other hand, an increased monitoring and regulating of individual bodies.[4] The ability to discuss mental illnesses such as depression openly and honestly has certainly helped many individuals seek treatment for serious problems. But, just as surely, the openness has also trained medical attention on individuals and behaviors once considered normal.[5] The development of new classes of antidepressants in the late 1980s led to new optimism about the treatment, even cure, of the illness. But, alongside the burgeoning pharmaceutical industry, an increased rhetorical production has fostered new practices of recognizing and responding to the self and its health and/or illness.

This talk and text reflects and helps construct the status of health in contemporary U.S. society. It requires practices of self-care, both self-regulating and self-doctoring behaviors such as the increased use of drugs and alternative therapies, and, also, potentially more rhetorically sophisticated responses as well. The language through which we experience and express our health (or illness) plays a crucial role in preparing our physical selves for medical intervention. This, then, is the power of such language: it can precipitate action by mapping the cognitive terrain and persuading us that we are (or are not) in need of treatment, and it can shape the forms of treatment to which we are willing to subject ourselves. To attend to the language of mental health and illness is to find oneself drawn into a series of debates, many of which are carried out in forms that leave unexamined the illness labels through which individuals struggle to define their lived experiences.

In recent bioethical and psychological scholarship, depression has become a focal point for arguments about "enhancement technologies," about the validity of various categories of mental illness, and about the medicalization of human emotion. In each of these debates, depression sometimes serves as a convenient example, but the definition of illness itself rarely receives clarification through such uses. For example, David Healey argues that antidepressants such as Prozac are "one of a growing number of agents that modulate lifestyles rather than cure diseases."[6] His argument directs attention toward the uses of antidepressant medications that respond to social rather than biological needs, and it therefore lays the foundation for a rhetorical examination of the production of such social needs. Nevertheless, Healey's focus does not specifically account for the rhetorical pressures that condition the prescription and ingestion of antidepressant medications. Similarly, Allan Horwitz and Jerome Wakefield's *The Loss of Sadness* suggests that "what our culture once viewed as a reaction to failed hopes and aspirations it now regards as psychiatric illness."[7] Horwitz and Wakefield's examination of the role of psychiatry in promoting this medicalization of sadness implies the power of rhetorical processes, but ultimately focuses primarily on the professional maneuvers that shape healthcare practices instead of on the specifics of the words and genres through which these maneuvers are communicated. Thus, until now, much of the language used about depression—language that is often metaphorical (as in the expression "the black dog of depression") and figurative (as in "the blues")—has gone unremarked and unexamined.[8] This is a significant oversight, since the structures of language fundamentally *shape*, rather than merely reflect, cultural assumptions. Recent studies have yet to produce an adequate account of the role of language in the processes of defining depression and shaping the illness identities available in the twenty-first century. This is my project in the following pages: to interrogate the rhetorical forms—the definitional words, metaphors, typical stories, and genres—through which depression is expressed, experienced, and treated in order to understand the gendered illness identities that are available for adoption and, perhaps, rhetorical adaptation.

Depression's Imperative: Self-Doctoring for Social Recognition

William Styron scorns the term *depression* as "a noun with a bland tonality and lacking any magisterial presence . . . a true wimp of a word for such a major illness."[9] Deriding the linguistic emasculation of depression (and perhaps betraying an anxiety about the potentially feminizing power of depression as it is currently constructed), Styron voices the common belief that language is simply a matter of vocabulary: replace the name and the illness will achieve appropriate recognition. By contrast, I understand *depression* as an organizing principle that subjects a range of symptoms and behaviors to increased scrutiny and medical intervention. Far from "lacking . . . presence," *depression*, via its rhetorical environment, acquires and maintains broad and permeable boundaries: for example, so-called normal grief over the death of a loved one may shade into depression if the symptoms persist long enough (over two months) or disrupt "social functioning" too much. This potential for slippage from grief to illness—a potential that is measured by standards articulated in terms such as "social functioning"—reinforces the need for close attention to the language that expresses affective experiences and performances of the self. Depression, as a constellation of textual, social, and gendered experiences, offers an important site for exploring the language of health care and the discursive shaping of illness identities. As I will discuss in more detail in chapter 3, the choice of terms for depression, especially the categorical terms *disease* and *illness*, is particularly fraught. Medical anthropologists and sociologists distinguish between *disease*, a biological malfunction, and *illness*, a social experience of the body, in order to analyze different cultural responses to health statuses. Because I am interested in the contemporary social construction of depression, I will refer to it as an *illness* rather than as a *disease*, and I intend to explore the rhetorical framework through which individuals interpret their affective experiences rather than the biological or neurochemical structures that may contribute to them.

Rhetoricians are philosophers as much as politicians. Despite the commonplace understanding of *rhetoric* as mere artful syntax or, worse, as crafty manipulation of ideas, the field itself has long attended to the available modes of information delivery. In the following pages, I explore the persuasive power of depression itself—not just for those who suffer from it, but for everyone who must live either within or against definitions of the illness. After all, not to be depressed is to recognize oneself outside the boundaries of mental illness and to maintain that location by constant monitoring and self-evaluation. The language of depression implicates both healthy and ill individuals, and it encourages particular orientations of the self and legitimizes patterns of gendered behavior that have physical and social ramifications. Depression is, therefore, a rhetorical illness; it functions persuasively in our collective and individual consciousness.

To argue that depression is a rhetorical illness is *not*, however, to suggest that it does not exist in tangible and often terrible form for those who experience it. Quite the contrary: depression would have very little rhetorical force if it did not exist as a condition that causes real suffering in the world. Nevertheless, the illness has generated so many voicings that it expands beyond the doctor's office and into everyday life. Some maladies—a broken bone or a viral or bacterial infection—live relatively constrained rhetorical lives within patient charts, perhaps inspiring a warning notice or cautionary exhortation, but rarely requiring continual monitoring because their boundaries and etiologies are reasonably straightforward. In the case of depression, however, the description of illness is both familiar and alien, inspiring conflicting responses and requiring consistent surveillance and intervention. Depression inspires self-doctoring through the textual responses it requires; attending to these responses offers an additional avenue for social and medical intervention into the illness and, it might be hoped, prevention of it.

At one time, the advice to "talk to your doctor" might have come from a friend or acquaintance; but since 1997, when the FDA changed its guidelines for the marketing of prescription pharmaceuticals, the exhortation has appeared more often as the refrain in advertisements describing illnesses and, of course, promoting their "cures." Such advertisements serve as a new form of patient education; they work to construct illness categories (Generalized Anxiety Disorder, Depression, and Premenstrual Dysphoric Disorder, for instance) that individuals are encouraged to recognize as descriptive of their own problematic identities. The command to consult one's doctor satisfies legal considerations—the treatments for these new illnesses require a prescription—but it also occasions new patterns of communication between doctor and patient. One is not meant simply to talk to one's doctor; one is meant to talk *about* the specific illnesses and the treatments offered in the advertisements. The stakes of such discursive representations are high: people respond with acts of self-doctoring, literally serving as their own doctors and, figuratively, performing acts of self-fashioning that help them accommodate social expectations for their gendered identities.

The language used to describe illnesses such as depression—not only direct-to-consumer marketing materials, but also government informational texts, news reports, memoirs, and newsletters—creates new, typically gendered, illness identities that entail significant self-doctoring practices for both healthy and ill individuals. These textual practices are the basis of a discourse of depression that regulates the cultural recognition, treatment, and attitudes toward the illness and its sufferers. The boundaries of depression (and of the gendered identities of those associated with it) are constructed and maintained through the language patterns and structures used to discuss them; the discourse of depression encourages and naturalizes practices of self-doctoring, including increased attention to diagnosis, monitoring, and intervention. To name depression a rhetorical illness is not at all to suggest that it is not real or consequential. Rather, it opens a new line of inquiry into the illness and the discourse that constitutes and grows from it.

Sampling the Discourse of Depression

Practices of self-doctoring gain legitimacy and urgency within the discourse of depression. It is my hope, however, that a critical rhetorical stance may encourage more complex responses to that discourse, responses that refuse to assume unreflectively the narrow illness identities currently available. Such self-care—in opposition to self-*doctoring*, which simply submits the self to medical intervention—results from an analysis of the rhetorical power of particular forms and configurations of language. In what follows, I explore the rhetorical formation of a self-doctoring drive and its effects on the gendered illness identities that attend depression, but I also seek opportunities to encourage a more robust form of self-care that recognizes the power of the discourse and encourages more complex health and illness identities within it.

The self-doctoring drive has become central to contemporary mental health and illness in part because of the effective marketing of psychopharmaceuticals to consumers. In the last two decades of the twentieth century, the three most popular selective serotonin reuptake inhibitor (SSRI) antidepressants—Prozac, Paxil, and Zoloft—were approved by the FDA for use in the United States. In 1993, Kramer's *Listening to Prozac* documented remarkable responses to Prozac among some of his patients. In 1997, the FDA relaxed restrictions on direct-to-consumer marketing of prescription pharmaceuticals, which led to the rapid deployment of a new form of public communication about illnesses and available treatments. These milestones mark high points in the popularity and ubiquity of chemical explanations for illnesses such as depression, one of the most identifiable features of "biological psychiatry." Shortly after the turn of the twenty-first century, however, enthusiasm about antidepressants was increasingly tempered by skeptical scientific reports. In 2004, acting in response to data that indicated increased tendencies toward suicide among adolescent users of SSRIs, the FDA required pharmaceutical companies to include a "black box warning" in their patient information for those drugs. In 2007, researchers conducting a meta-analysis of drug trial information collected by the FDA concluded that, for all but the most severely depressed, SSRIs were no better than placebos in treating depression.[10] The decade 1995–2005 thus represents a moment in the history of depression when biological psychiatry offered the most productive models for the identification and treatment of the illness.

Exploring the discourse of depression in that decade, I turn to a range of public texts, including items as ephemeral as billboards and cartoons and as popular as memoirs, self-help texts, and direct-to-consumer advertisements. In addition, I work from a collection of texts representing accessible public knowledge of depression in the forms of news sources, government information materials, and a comprehensive run of a *Psychology Today* newsletter on depression. This corpus offers a synchronic view of the language that encourages self-doctoring as a response to depression and the gendered illness identities it entails. It is a systematic collection of texts: articles from *Newsweek* and the *New York Times*; selections from the depression newsletter, *Blues Buster*; and documents published by the National Institute of Mental Health (NIMH). These texts represent the public knowledge of depression as it has been collected, synthesized, and published by powerful social institutions.

For samples of news discourse, I used the full-text database Lexis-Nexis to search *Newsweek* and the *New York Times* from January 1, 1995, through December 31, 2005. The resulting articles were narrowed by excluding those that had only a passing reference to the disorder (e.g., an article in *Newsweek* that addressed infertility with only two instances of the word "depression"). This process resulted in a total of 147 articles, 81 from *Newsweek* (63,450 words) and 66 from the *New York Times* (62,380 words). To this collection, I added representative text samples from the entire print run of the newsletter *Blues Buster* (July 2001 through May 2004): the lead story of each issue, the "Action Strategies" section of advice for intervention, and the final question and answer feature. These three sections, totaling 84 separate items (88,550 words), provide a cross-section of the types of text in the newsletter. To incorporate government public service material, I selected NIMH documents on depression published or revised after 2000 (8 texts, 18,868 words). In total, my computer-analyzable collection comprises 239 articles and 238,035 words.

To this corpus, I added first-person memoirs of depression published in the same general time frame. I chose five single-author texts written by men, five written by women, and four multi-authored collections or studies that included multiple voices from individuals suffering from depression. Men's experiences of depression are represented by William Styron's classic text *Darkness Visible* (1990), David Karp's *Speaking of Sadness: Depression, Disconnection, and the Meaning of Illness* (1996), Jeffery Smith's *Where the Roots Reach for Water: A Personal and Natural History of Melancholia* (1999), Lewis Wolpert's *Malignant Sadness: The Anatomy of Depression* (1999), and Andrew Solomon's *The Noonday Demon: An Atlas of Depression* (2001). Women's experiences are detailed in Elizabeth Wurtzel's *Prozac Nation: A Memoir* (1994), Martha Manning's *Undercurrents* (1995), Tracy Thompson's *The Beast: A Journey Through Depression* (1996), Lauren Slater's *Prozac Diary* (1998), and Meri Nana-Ama Danquah's *Willow Weep for Me: A Black Woman's Journey through Depression* (1999). Finally, multivocal texts included Kathy Cronkite's *On the Edge of Darkness: Conversations about Conquering Depression* (1994), Nell Casey's edited collection *Unholy Ghost: Writers on Depression* (2001), Lauren Dockett's *The Deepest Blue: How Women Face and Overcome Depression* (2001), and David Karp's *Is It Me or My Meds?* (2006). Collectively these texts, though edited and therefore potentially subject to the conventions and narrative expectations of their contexts of publication, offer longer explorations of depression and its associated identities than news articles possibly can. In addition, these texts are often recommended to and by depression sufferers as forms of comfort, identification, and self-help.

Analysis of printed texts remains, however, a relatively two-dimensional representation of the language of illness. To complement this analysis, I conducted three semistructured group interviews. In 2002, I spoke with two groups of women about their experiences with and understandings of depression. The interviews were designed as small group discussions to focus on forms of conversation as much as on the content of the talk. The women spoke to one another as well as to me, and these interactions reveal collective pressures toward self-doctoring that mirror those identified in the discourse at large. Seven women participated; each was experiencing mild to moderate symptoms of depression, as measured by the National Institute of Mental Health's CES-D index.[11] As members of the "worried well," they represent a primary target for information and pharmaceutical marketing campaigns.[12] The women in my interviews were students at a large research university: about half were undergraduates (four) and the other half were graduate students (three). They ranged in ages from about nineteen to thirty-five, and were white (four) and Asian American (three); they did not know one another before the interviews took place. I digitally recorded and transcribed each ninety-minute group interview, and all transcripts included here use pseudonyms and generalized details (e.g., "humanities major") to protect the identities of the participants. My own initials (KE) are used to identify me in excerpts from the interviews.

The first group interview included four women: Paige, who had just finished her humanities undergraduate degree; Claire, a graduate student in the humanities; Su-Ting, a graduate student in the health sciences; and Tiffany, a senior undergraduate in the humanities. The second group included Mei, a senior undergraduate in the health sciences; Jennifer, a graduate student in the natural sciences; and Stephanie, an undergraduate in the humanities. A third interview, also in 2002, included four mental health professionals who provided a sample of professional talk within the discourse of depression. These women were recruited from a university environment and were all finished or nearly finished with their advanced degrees. This group included Laurie, a psychologist; Ellen, a psychiatrist; Joan, a social worker; and Betty, a psychiatric nurse. In all of my interviews, I used an ethnographic methodology to gather demographic and situational information from the women.[13] This interview process makes use of the individuals' own terms and conceptual frameworks to describe their situations and experiences. Thus, the conversations of these groups of women provide an important balance to my analysis of news and public informational texts about depression. These conversations provide evidence of the persuasive power of the discourse that both defines and resists defining depression too narrowly at the turn of the twenty-first century. They also suggest moments when individuals can challenge the discourse and make personal use of the language through which they must experience and express their health and illness.

Within the contemporary discourse of depression, a variety of rhetorical structures—the definitions, metaphors, stories and stock characters, and genres that I will describe below—encourage practices of self-doctoring that orchestrate the submission of the self to medical and chemical interventions. While these may be appropriate treatments in some cases, they have been accepted by a wide population and without much challenge (until recently) from other discourses of mental health.[14] As a response, I argue for counterstrategies that enact a rhetorical care of the self, which critically engages with the discourses of mental health in order to revitalize a dialogic negotiation of health and illness identities. Through such counterstrategies, practices of *care* might, I hope, be substituted for those of *doctoring* that currently prevail.

The chapters that follow explore structural phenomena within the discourse of depression to provide a more nuanced explanation of practices of self-doctoring that individuals are compelled to perform. Across a wide range of rhetorical situations, these chapters expose the discursive construction of the gendered self and the direction of self-doctoring energies toward maintaining women's emotional and men's professional identities. Chapter 1 investigates the rhetorical nature of depression, arguing that depression's deep embedding within language makes it an important site for exploring the construction of gendered health and illness identities. Chapter 2 describes in more detail the role of language in supporting biological psychiatry at the turn of the twenty-first century, in promoting practices of self-doctoring, and in offering opportunities for a rhetorical care of the self. In the next four chapters, the analysis attends to specific structural features within the discourse of depression.

Examining depression through linguistic patterns of its definition, I argue in chapter 3 that such patterns compel readers toward practices of self-doctoring because the precise measurement of depression remains elusive. The chapter begins with an analysis of the frequency of the categorical terms: *disease*, *disorder*, *illness*, and *condition*, then moves outward to examine the definitional moments in memoirs and other texts. This analysis documents the development of depression as not just an illness, but as a *woman's* illness. Chapters 4 and 5 address rhetorical structures—metaphor and narrative—that work to establish the boundaries and expected activities of healthy and ill selves. In chapter 4 I collect and analyze the prevalent metaphors for depression and the depressed self, including biological-mechanical metaphors that accompany the "chemical imbalance" etiology for depression; spatial metaphors, such as the common description of depression as "an abyss"; bestial metaphors such as the "black dog"; and literate metaphors that return to the themes of an intensely rhetorical illness. Working from recent research on the cognitive functions of metaphor, I argue that these metaphors portray the depressed individual as an isolated and gendered figure whose identity becomes inseparable from the illness itself. This isolation encourages narrow practices of self-doctoring based on notions of a faulty neurological self. Nevertheless, some metaphors for depression, particularly those that emphasize literate and semiotic communication, seem to work against monological responses, opening spaces and opportunities for a rhetorical care of the self.

Building on notions of dialogue that are introduced by these metaphors of communication, in chapter 5 I argue for narrative and rhetorical competencies as responses to the discourse of depression. The characters and plots contained within stories of depression create prototypical depression sufferers, and they encode a series of gendered messages about living with the illness. Within such stories, an economy of emotion and a series of gendered social networks take shape and encourage individuals to render themselves visible within each through the citation of key plots and characters. Thus, chapters 4 and 5 work together to explore the persuasive appeals within the discourse of depression that operate primarily through display—through the praise and blame of exemplary individuals and experiences[15]—and which help compel reciprocal displays of gendered illness identities by individuals themselves.

Chapter 6 begins with the genre of the self-diagnostic quiz as a means of defining depression and the gendered self. Making use of recent work in rhetorical genre theory, which holds that genres are social actions rather than static forms, I argue that the widespread use of this genre contributes to the gendering of the illness both because its form aligns closely with women's self-help genres and because its content skews symptoms of depression toward stereotypically feminine experiences. Further, as rhetorical genre theory predicts, the symptoms list reconfigures the social interactions between doctors and patients. Inviting users to diagnose themselves, the genre performs as a referring physician, challenging the traditional authority vested in primary care doctors. In this reorientation of actors, individuals, and especially women whose use of the genre is conditioned by their familiarity with similar forms, quite literally doctor themselves. Thus, the symptoms list organizes and facilitates narrow practices of self-doctoring, centered on diagnosis and resulting very often in the prescription of psychopharmaceuticals.

The conclusion to this project revisits the situation of the self as both subject to and the subject of the discourse of depression, arguing that in a world saturated with the terms and conditions of diagnosis, practices of self-doctoring have come to be primary in the performance of identity. Returning to the assumption of a consumer empowered through discourse, I argue that, rather than empowerment, individuals are more likely to find only a narrow range of responses to their illness experiences. As a counterstrategy to such limited practices of self-doctoring, I borrow from multiple disciplines to imagine a series of dialogical tactics that might promote a rhetorical care of the self. Opening the opportunity for dialogic uses of the discourse of depression, in the conclusion I argue that better health care must be predicated not simply on an *understanding* of the discursive construction of gendered illness identities, but also on the promotion of individuals' *rhetorical uses* of such constructions.

1

Depression, a Rhetorical Illness

It is a double cruelty that depression often silences its sufferers. Beyond its affective pain, whether the illness manifests as a withdrawal from social interaction or as a permanent physical escape via suicide, individuals experiencing the symptoms of depression often seem to have limited linguistic resources available to them.[1] According to many sufferers, words cannot describe the pain of depression, and yet it is ironically a condition largely known through the words that they do find. Access to treatment occurs *only* through the interpretive act of diagnosis, and diagnosis itself depends on the report of recognizable symptoms. The patterns of expression through which individuals articulate their experiences as, for example, matters of brain chemistry, fundamentally shape their ideas of health and illness. Collectively, these patterns constitute a "discourse of depression," which exceeds the utterance of any one statement, but which is also reiterated within each statement. In other words, to recognize a particular string of words as referring to or explaining depression, speakers draw on a collective memory that results from repeated patterns of articulation. In the act of recognition, speakers and hearers validate and perpetuate the discourse's structuring power.

As language scholars have long recognized, the words in which ideas are presented are not neutral; they fundamentally shape the entities to which they refer. While notions of strong linguistic determinism have been discredited, the operation of linguistic relativity—the idea that language, as a cultural phenomenon, does influence thought and behavior—forms the basis for much social critique. Studies in language and gender in the 1970s and 1980s, for example, demonstrated the nonuniversality of ostensibly neutral nouns and pronouns such as "man" and "he"—in research that asked individuals to locate pictures to represent "chairman" (which collected largely male images) and "chairperson" (which collected mixed sex images)—despite the then-current arguments that masculine terms were always assumed to be inclusive. As a result of these analyses and the awareness campaigns they launched, public discourse has shifted toward more self-consciously "gender-neutral" discursive practices.[2] For studies of medical language, this case is instructive, cautioning against contemporary beliefs that assume neutrality within diagnostic labels. Indeed, as the historian Laura Hirschbein has pointed out, as early as the 1970s, "the supposition that depression was a disease of women had become entrenched to the point that studies done entirely on women were presented as studies on depression itself."[3] Underlying beliefs about depression may lead researchers to make assumptions about both the illness and the identities attached to it. Compiling research on depression that fails to account for the necessarily gendered identities of sufferers ignores differences in socialization and emotional expression between men and women. Such generalized results then perpetuate the assumption that depression is a woman's illness, because women are most likely to be recognizable in the research results.

In much the same way, the construction of symptom statements—for example, "excessive crying"—has material effects on which individuals receive diagnoses and, consequently, treatments. Such symptom statements rely on assumptions about gender and about depression embedded in the discourse. What constitutes *excessive* crying? The answer depends on normalized emotional responses, and a judgment of excess results at least in part from comparison to the reports of research studies such as those Hirschbein critiques for their gender bias. The contemporary discursive landscape of depression is increasingly dominated by corporate pharmaceutical interests, whose powerful marketing machines have supported a proliferation of new disease entities.[4] Such new diseases are represented to us through language designed to mask gendered assumptions and to appeal to the broadest possible audiences. This language is predicated on the close association between disease and its particular pharmaceutical remedy, as Andrew Lakoff succinctly describes the equation: "'depression' should be treatable by an 'anti-depressant.'"[5] The logic—encoded in the simplicity of the prefix *anti*—excludes myriad additional mechanisms and circumstances that might affect the experience and treatment of depression. In response, the tools of rhetorical analysis offer important counterstrategies for maintaining a complex, situationally sensitive knowledge of health and illness.

To suggest that language and rhetorical analysis might materially affect the experience of depression is to accept what humanities scholars have labeled the "linguistic turn," whereby *discourse* takes on a specific critical meaning, and objective reality is available only through the nonneutral mediation of language. *Discourse*, following Michel Foucault, refers to the collection of statements a culture makes about a given subject within a particular historical moment. Foucault argues that cultural concepts such as *madness* are iteratively defined via the statements—linguistic, institutional, and even geographical—that are made about them. Physical structures attached to madness—the asylums, social welfare programs, and penitentiaries—give concrete form to the attitudes encoded in the language used to describe it. At any given time, Foucault argues, the discursive construction of an entity such as madness gives rise to the corresponding social responses to it, ranging from tolerance to incarceration.[6] In the seventeenth and eighteenth centuries, the move from communal treatment of the mentally ill to institutional treatment and then to asylum treatment can be seen not only in medical practice, but also in medical rhetoric; in the twentieth century, the rapid deinstitutionalization of the mentally ill appears natural and inevitable due to another change in medical rhetoric. Discourse, then, refers to the accumulation and organization of linguistic and social responses to and configurations of a concept such as depression, and this accumulation shapes future interactions with the concept. Depression becomes recognizable *as illness* through discourse, and the discourse of depression is continually shaped by ongoing experiences of the illness.

Concretely, the contemporary discourse of depression comprises all utterances currently recognizable as referring to the illness. The discourse sanctions and categorizes such utterances; thus, we understand the phrase "chemical imbalance" as a scientific explanation for depression, but the phrase "under the influence of Saturn" as only a poetic allusion. The regulatory function of discourse operates through the accretion of multiple utterances, but it can be, to some extent, dissected into its component structures. For example, the definitions, metaphors, stories, and genres through which depression may be expressed each contribute to the metastructure of the discourse. Individually, these components encourage particular practices of self-doctoring; together, they reinforce the dominance of biological psychiatry and the gendered identities available to sufferers. Thus, the "discourse of depression" refers to the normative power of the collection of linguistic structures and rhetorical appeals that characterize talk and text about the illness. For analytical convenience, I have divided the discourse into the four components—definitions, metaphors, stories, and genres—though there are certainly other possible divisions. A rhetorical care of the self, as opposed to uncritical self-doctoring, requires attention to these and other layers of discourse in order to open avenues for critique and meaningful social action.

Scholars in critical discourse analysis, a combination of critical sociology and applied linguistics, direct such attention toward such specific language structures in order to understand the functioning of social power. Focusing on the internal features and organization of texts as well as on the interactions between texts and the social scenes in which they are embedded, critical discourse analysis offers a model that accounts for the effects of language within the social, material world. The late twentieth and early twenty-first centuries have been characterized as a period of significant social, linguistic, and economic fluidity. Lilie Chouliaraki and Norman Fairclough claim that one of the signal characteristics of this "late modern" era is the rapid production and circulation of texts about concrete realities and processes. Such texts— collectively, a series of discourses such as those of medicine, industrialization, or globalization—both structure and are structured by their contextual realities. Chouliaraki and Fairclough write that "an important characteristic of the economic, social and cultural changes of late modernity [is] that they exist as *discourses* as well as processes that are taking place outside discourse, and that the processes that are taking place outside discourse are substantively shaped by those discourses."[7] In other words, late modernity is saturated with textuality—perhaps even more so than other periods due to the rapid proliferation of communication technologies—organizing texts around activities and activities around texts. In the legal world, for example, a death sentence (a text) cannot become an execution (an action) without a warrant (another text), which legitimizes a homicide (a different action) by reframing it within a judicial code (a larger text). Thus, as Chouliaraki and Fairclough write, "Discourse is a form of power, a mode of formation of beliefs/values/desires, an institution, a mode of social relating, a material practice. Conversely, power, social relations, material practices, institutions, beliefs, etc. are in part discourse."[8] In the social scene of mental illness, discourse shapes the possible interactions among patients, doctors, caregivers, and other actors. The accumulation of statements, physical practices, technologies, and geographies of mental illness call into being the depressed individual by representing an expected orientation to a gendered self.

DEPRESSION IS a rhetorical illness. Our comprehension and experience of it starts from and returns to the language we have available to describe it. Further, the future research and clinical practices that may develop in response to depression are shaped by the same conceptual discourse that frames our contemporary cultural attitudes toward the illness. Within the discourse of depression, a variety of rhetorical structures reflect and privilege the vocabulary of biological psychiatry and the conceptual model it encodes. For individuals, a logical response includes various discursive and material practices of self-doctoring. These practices, however, reinforce individuals' isolation and ignore additional discursive and material responses that may afford a more complex understanding of gender, the self, and mental health.

The current character of depression's rhetoricity—situated within the scientific frame of biological psychiatry and reinforcing the discursive mandate for self-doctoring—encourages individuals to monitor their affective experiences closely and to suspect their brain chemistry when those experiences do not meet expectations. Nevertheless, this rhetoricity might inaugurate a curiosity characteristic of a rhetorical care of the self rather than the acceptance characteristic of self-doctoring. Indeed, dissatisfactions with contemporary models and revelations of adverse events associated with antidepressants seem to be surfacing as rhetorical challenges to the supremacy of purely biochemical interventions. A rhetorical care of the self does not deny the potential effectiveness of such interventions, but it encourages more dialogue about illness and its social, gendered environments, rather than more talk about symptoms that have been isolated from their contexts. Pedagogical support for the rhetorical care of the self—including additional interdisciplinary activities that promote critical reading strategies—might encourage individuals to seek and receive a variety of appropriate treatments. Such treatments may include psychotropic medications, but they may also include the development of new social institutions and practices aimed at integrating rather than isolating individuals.

The broad themes of definition, self, and gender arc through the discourse of depression, each coming to rest in individual texts and then returning to circulation in future utterances. The individual subject who emerges within this textual landscape cannot help but acquire the gendered meanings attached to the illness identity. The discourse, quite simply, renders audible only those patients who speak the right language from within the expected selves. In the current literary and nonfictional environment, the proliferation of available texts for analysis provides a rich opportunity to draw attention to the linguistic structures that characterize the discourse of depression and that construct the illness within a biomedical model. Individual practices of self-doctoring emerge and take shape as responses to the discursive pressures to maintain one's health or, at the very least, treat one's illness(es).

Depression is a rhetorical phenomenon in three distinct senses. First, it is an illness saturated with language; it inspires nearly compulsive storytelling. Such extensive talk not only shapes the illness and social responses to it, but it also inspires the judgment encoded in the phrases such as Solomon's "everyone and his uncle Bob," who tell of their experiences with the illness. The implied redundancy of "Uncle Bob's" talk about his illness stands in for contradictory rhetorical impulses both to narrate and to silence illness experiences. In this way, depression is a rhetorical phenomenon because it inhabits a familiar place in social conversation. In addition to this storytelling, diagnosis of depression relies heavily on the precise language of symptoms. Self- and peer-reporting of these symptoms adopt the patterns of articulation common to the circulating discourse; in other words, symptoms described in individuals' stories become models for future descriptions of others' illness experiences. Thus, depression is recognized through repeated rhetorical patterns of reference. Finally, depression serves as a model against which other behavior is read. Within the stories we tell of depression are messages about what a "good" or "normal" person looks, acts, and feels like. Thus, talk about depression frames the illness itself—both what gets recognized as depression (sadness, disengagement, loss of pleasure) and what gets ignored (violence, sociopathic behavior)—while simultaneously reinforcing norms about emotion, social functioning, and gender roles.

Compulsive Storytelling: Authoring the Prozac Nation

The discourse of depression draws heavily on pharmaceutical interventions that seem to promise simple cures. The historically recent and relatively unprecedented popular use of psychotropic drugs serves as an indication of our collective entry into what Lawrence Rubin calls "the new asylum," a place where the walls of confinement are invisible and where "it has become difficult to know where mental health ends and mental illness begins."[9] Drug companies and popular culture more widely have manufactured this "Psychotropia," where the blurring of boundaries makes every individual a potential patient.[10] Clearly, direct-to-consumer advertising contributes to the formation of this new asylum, but it is only one factor in a larger discourse of mental health and illness. In the case of depression, a variety of rhetorical practices have contributed to a sense of ubiquity and nearly universal vulnerability. Popular films and television series refer to antidepressants by brand name; personal Web sites and blogs profess faith in or poke fun at the latest treatments; memoirs and biographies detail talk therapies, prescriptions, and hospitalizations; casual conversations become the basis for pharmaceutical requests. Depression has become, according to one popular mental health Web site, "the common cold of mental disorders."[11] This phrase encodes attitudes toward the illness and its sufferers that indicate both universality and triviality. Much like the reference to "everyone and his uncle Bob" experiencing depression, this phrase indicates a blasé acceptance of the illness's presence that would have been unthinkable only a few decades ago. In my interview with the mental health professionals, Joan, a master of social work student in her late twenties, discloses that nearly a quarter of her acquaintances are taking antidepressants. This number does not surprise her colleagues in the interview—just a moment earlier, Laurie, a clinical psychologist, had noted that twenty-one of eighty students in one of her classes raised their hands when she asked how many were taking Prozac—but the comfort with disclosing and discussing depression seems to be a generational difference among the mental health professionals. Joan is at least fifteen years younger than Laurie, and her acquaintances' forthright discussion of their medication use is praised by Laurie and the other mental health professionals for opening new narrative territory.

As talk and text about antidepressants becomes commonplace, the drugs themselves form the basis of new communicative strategies—they encapsulate social attitudes, encouraging individuals to take on new identities as they take in the medications. The most famous of the antidepressants is, of course, Eli Lilly's Prozac, which was the first of the SSRIs to be approved by the FDA, in 1987. Technologically and rhetorically, Prozac enacts new patterns of communication. In one scholarly collection of essays, Prozac is described as having "moved out of the doctor's office and into the culture as a whole."[12] Indeed, the brand name has been used by memoirists and scholars alike as a metonym for depression itself and for the illness (and treatment) experiences. A brief tour of recent book titles demonstrates its currency, both in autobiographical writing—*Prozac Diary*, *Prozac Highway*—and in scholarly and cultural critique: *Listening to Prozac*, *Prozac on the Couch*, *Let Them Eat Prozac*, *Prozac as a Way of Life*, *Prozac Backlash*.[13] Across these titles and within these works, the cultural concept of *Prozac* inspires authorship and also authors new social interactions. Lauren Slater's "Prozac Doctor," to whom she is referred for her prescription, has lost his identifying features, just as the public—the "them" in David Healy's *Let Them Eat Prozac*—has been reduced to passive and interchangeable consumers of medical technologies. We seem to live, not simply in Psychotropia, but in a "Prozac Nation," to borrow the title of Elizabeth Wurtzel's bestselling memoir of her experiences with depression.

The rhetorical landscape of depression is, at times, indistinguishable from the topography of medication, and this confusion is at least in part a product of the discourse of depression. Toward the end of her memoir, Wurtzel comments, anxiously:

> "I can't escape the icky feeling I get every time I'm sitting in a full car and everyone but the driver is on Prozac. I can't get away from some sense that after years of trying to get people to take depression seriously—of saying, I have a *disease*, I *need* help—now it has gone beyond the point of recognition as a real problem to become something that appears totally trivial. . . . After all, the media phenomenon of Prozac is such that it's turning a serious problem into a joke at a point when that really should not be happening: By most accounts, two-thirds of the people with severe depression are not being treated for it. And they are the ones who are likely to get lost in the rhetoric."[14]

Blaming the popularity and ubiquity of Prozac—both as a term signifying a whole constellation of health-care practices and as a signifier of business interests in those same practices—Wurtzel draws attention to the human consequence of muddled definition. Worrying about "the ones who are likely to get lost in the rhetoric," Wurtzel reminds us that individuals can indeed become so embedded in discourse as to become invisible. The proliferation and diffusion of meanings attached to Prozac threaten to overwhelm serious illness identities with simplified pharmaceutical solutions, which, when they are not immediately successful, leave sufferers without alternative stories to tell.

In another memoir, Martha Manning notes this rhetorical reduction. "People," she writes, "seem to be more forthright these days about discussing depression. Things have loosened up, even talking about medicine. Hell, the cashier in the grocery store told me yesterday that she's on Prozac."[15] Here, talk about Prozac amounts to talk about depression, and the quotidian scene of the supermarket, paired with Manning's interjection "hell," reinforces a sense that the discursive location of depression has become both commonplace and inextricable from its treatment. Strong ties between illness and treatment artificially collapse the distances between these experiences, emptying the discourse of possible alternative responses. More talk is not inherently a bad thing, but the contemporary talk of medication reflects new mediations of the self via pharmaceuticals, and, importantly, via *talk about* pharmaceuticals. Both Wurtzel and Manning express frustration over illness identities that are trivialized by the vernacular popularity of Prozac.

The consequences of living in a "Prozac Nation" are both rhetorical and material, and the language surrounding depression is more than a reflection of these new realities. Prozac stands in for all recent antidepressants as the cultural icon for a desire to feel "better than well."[16] Depression and the contemporary modes of its treatment have occasioned new discursive practices that not only shape experiences of the illness, but that also encourage the growth of self-doctoring, which includes both an impulse to self-diagnose and also a significant monitoring and manipulation of the "self" to comply with social and emotional expectations. Such self-doctoring works to align individuals with the regimes of biological psychiatry and to marginalize the social matrix that comes to serve as merely a canvas for self-articulations.

Despite the mass of readily available information about the illness, Lewis Wolpert writes in his memoir that "it would be misleading to say that depression is understood."[17] This lack of clarity appears, however, as much a matter of discursive construction as does the illness identity itself. Informative texts, ostensibly provided to help consumers make educated decisions about their treatment options, often further confuse the thresholds between everyday experiences and medical symptoms. A constant refrain in many of these texts is: Talk to your doctor. Commanding the production of *more* language about depression, this refrain satisfies the legal requirements for obtaining medical advice and prescription medications, but it also signals to individuals that *they* have something to say about the illness. It promises to give individuals a sense of their own subjectivity, even though to take up this advice is already to have (at least partially) accepted the biochemical illness identity itself. The exhortation rests on the medical assumption that consultation will produce diagnosis, diagnosis will produce treatment (especially via pharmaceuticals), and treatment will produce health. To accept the illness identity offered in these texts is to place oneself on this particular trajectory. But before patients fill their Prozac prescriptions, they must first recognize themselves and their experiences as conforming to the prevailing articulation of depression. They do this largely through their interactions with texts: self-diagnostic quizzes, conversations with friends, memoirs and self-help books, Web sites and government guidelines. Thus, rhetorical intervention precedes medical intervention, and even the medical intervention comes first in the form of language.

The Rhetoric of the *DSM*

The American Psychiatric Association's *Diagnostic and Statistical Manual of Mental Disorders* (the *DSM*) functions as a master genre that coordinates much of the discourse of depression. It occupies the rarefied and rarely questioned position of an objective reference tool, somehow escaping the bounds of its all-too-human authorship. [18] In the words of Robert Spitzer, "The very success of the *DSM* and its descriptive criteria at a practical level has allowed the field of psychiatry [and, indeed, the public in general] to ignore some basic conceptual issues . . . especially the question of how to distinguish disorder from normal suffering."[19] Spitzer's critique—important because it comes from the man who, in his own words, "formulated the definitions of mental disorder in the introductions to the *DSM-III*, the *DSM-III-R* . . . and the *DSM-IV*, which aim to explain the reasons that certain conditions were included in and other types of problems excluded from the *Manual*"—opens a space for a close analysis of the rhetorical history of the *DSM*.[20] Such an analysis models one strategic intervention into the discourse of depression: it encourages individuals to consider the purposes of the *DSM* and to resituate depression within a complex rhetorical scene, rather than at the nexus of brain chemistry and psychopharmacology. Highlighting the disparate goals of psychiatric *research* and clinical *treatment* that influenced the creation of the *DSM*, a historical critique reveals that illness categories serve a variety of purposes, not all of which benefit the individuals experiencing the symptoms that these categories assemble.

The *DSM-I*, published in 1952, and all of its successors contain various disclaimers, centering on the uneasy alliance between psychiatric research and clinical treatment. In the words of Gerald Klerman, "Medicine studies diseases, but treats patients."[21] Standard psychiatric nomenclature grew out of a need for statistical record-keeping data, and, in 1917, the APA adopted "a plan for uniform statistics in hospitals for mental disease."[22] This original goal—the collection of consistent numerical data—only uncomfortably aligns with the work of clinicians, whose primary attention rests in the individual circumstances of patients. Indeed, one foundational study of the rhetoric of mental health records warns that "all writers and readers of mental health records . . . should understand that the *DSM* language system . . . governs clinical diagnostics, assessments, evaluations, and recommendations . . . according to a system that was not originally designed for that purpose at all, but, rather, for national data collection."[23] This exhortation—that we understand the poor fit between the original vocabulary of data collection and its current placement in the diagnostic manual—is a call for a critical stance toward the genre systems of mental health care. It requires readers to practice a *rhetorical* care of the self.

A look at the historical versions of the *DSM* provides a place to ground such a critical stance. The *DSM-I* (1952) acknowledges the disparate goals—those of data collection and those of clinical use—that coexist uneasily in the document itself. *DSM-I* cautions that clinical treatment will require additional information beyond what is needed for a diagnosis to be counted in epidemiological figures: "The mere stating of the diagnosis (including its qualifying terms) is not sufficient for certain conditions, since it does not furnish enough information to describe the clinical picture."[24] Nevertheless, subsequent revisions of the *DSM* distance themselves from this problematic differentiation between *research* and *clinical* uses of the nomenclature. In *DSM-II* (1968), under the subtitle "The Recording of Diagnoses," readers are cautioned that "every attempt has been made to express the diagnoses in the clearest and simplest terms possible within the framework of modern usage. Clinicians will significantly improve communication and research by recording their diagnoses in the same terms."[25] By 1980 and the publication of *DSM-III*, the value of clinical judgment has been nearly subsumed into the project of research validity: the *DSM-III* "reflects an increased commitment . . . to reliance on data as the basis for understanding mental disorders."[26] Starting with the *DSM-III*, an explicit statement of the document's purpose "to provide clear descriptions of diagnostic categories in order to enable clinicians and investigators to diagnose, communicate about, study, and treat various mental disorders" appears in each introduction. [27] And, while the *DSM-III-R* (1987) cautions that such descriptions are "only an initial step in a comprehensive evaluation," neither it nor the *DSM-IV* (1994) nor the most recent revision, the *DSM-IV-TR* (2000) acknowledges the roots of *DSM* descriptions in practices of data collection separate from clinical treatment. [28] Tracing, as this brief overview begins to do, the discursive "forgetting" of the *DSM*'s origins in epidemiology encourages a critical distance that may allow readers (and mental health professionals) to orient themselves as tactical users of such texts rather than as practitioners narrowly bound by its authority.

Beyond attending to the origins of the *DSM*, a critical intervention into the system of mental health expertise includes investigating the means by which the document itself organizes narrow practices of self-doctoring. The *DSM* encourages extensive self- and other-monitoring: clinical judgment must often rely on "information from family members and other third parties (in addition to the individual) regarding the individual's performance."[29] Here, the "performance" of the individual is subject to monitoring by a variety of others, and the individual's own assessment is relegated to a parenthetical inclusion. Performances, after all, require audiences, and the self becomes vulnerable to the observations of "other third parties." Nevertheless, the individual's own reports are important for diagnosis, and the monitoring of the self becomes a key factor in maintaining mental health and identifying mental illness. As individuals traverse the health and illness identities available to them, they are encouraged to compare their experiences to standards such as those contained in the *DSM*.

Nevertheless, the *DSM* does appear to understand its task not simply as scientific, but as rhetorical as well. In the introduction, the authors describe their goals of making the manual "practical and useful for clinicians by striving for brevity of criteria sets, clarity of language, and explicit statements of the constructs embodied in the diagnostic criteria."[30] In this statement, the authors acknowledge that the mental disorders they describe are *constructs*, that they are foundationally rhetorical, given shape through the descriptive phrases that surround them. The desire to provide "clarity of language" is, of course, the desire to shed the influence of this rhetoric, to find objective and transferable words with which to construct disorders. This desire inhabits the calls for "brevity" and "explicit statements," both of which attempt to limit the extent of language interference. The manual is wary of the language it is obliged to use; it attempts to restrict that language as much as possible, but the possibility for additional interpretations remains.

The attempts to restrict language hope to control the application of the *DSM* as much as they do to confine the meanings of the words that constitute it. The *DSM-IV-TR* sets up a curiously suspicious stance toward its audience. The authors caution that the "specific diagnostic criteria included . . . are meant to serve as guidelines to be informed by clinical judgment and are not meant to be used in a cookbook fashion." It thus warns practitioners to apply sound judgment, which may mean departing from a strict interpretation of the criteria listed in the manual, yet in another place, it warns practitioners to avoid "excessively flexible and idiosyncratic application" of the criteria.[31] In both cases, users are expected to become their own monitors, they must discipline their actions according to the norms of their profession, while the text that outlines these norms continues to evince anxiety about the illness borders it polices. At least part of the anxiety of self-monitoring arises from the *DSM's* position as intermediary between two professional communities. The manual is meant "to facilitate research and improve communication among clinicians and researchers."[32] A primary emphasis on research shapes the translation between researchers and clinicians, recalling traditional academic divisions between the "makers of new knowledge" (researchers) and the practitioners who apply it (clinicians). These tensions exist in most academic disciplines, but in the *DSM-IV-TR* the suspicion of practitioners expressed via language such as "cookbook fashion" and "idiosyncratic application" makes the process of diagnosis itself seem more art than science, even though the goal is ostensibly pure, objective science (via research). In this foundational document, disease definitions are potentially subject to user error and are therefore in need of constant monitoring.

In the case of "Major Depressive Disorder," the *DSM* language requires surveillance of the self as a logical response to an individualized scale of symptom severity. In the text description that accompanies the checklist of symptoms, the manual suggests that diagnosis will vary from case to case. It cautions that an episode "must be accompanied by clinically significant distress or impairment in social, occupational, or other important areas of functioning" in order to qualify for diagnosis. The very next sentence, however, redefines "impairment": "For some individuals with milder episodes, functioning may appear to be normal but requires markedly increased effort."[33] This hedging around the quality of an individual's "functioning"—which may either cause "clinically significant distress" or "appear to be normal"—allows for individualized assessments, and therefore relies on the subjective reports of patients and their acquaintances, and the judgments of clinicians. In addition, the description focuses on community and social functioning, including productivity in the workplace, which further encourages self-monitoring and self-modeling toward social expectations. Depression, then, becomes visible only when an individual does not produce or interact as expected.

Among the nine criteria of depression, three may be established by "subjective report" or "observation made by others" (depressed mood, diminished interest or pleasure in activities, diminished ability to think or concentrate) and a fourth may be met only if "observed by others" (psychomotor agitation or retardation). These modes of ascertaining symptoms direct attention to the self and its interactions, and they involve individuals and their close acquaintances in their own diagnoses. Despite this invitation to participate, only one of the nine criteria includes an explicit measure with which to determine the severity of an experience—"a change of more than 5% of body weight in a month"—and even this criterion is not absolute, since it can additionally be met by a "decrease or increase in appetite." Similarly, the possibility of opposite affective experiences—*decreases* or *increases* in appetite, *in*somnia or *hyper*somnia, psychomotor *agitation* or *retardation*—fulfilling the same criteria helps to enlarge the population to whom the diagnosis may apply and also to implicate a wide range of behavior and experience as potential symptoms of illness. Patients' and others' subjective reports, used as evidence for diagnosis, participate in the circulating discourse of depression. These reports reflect the available language about depression: direct-to-consumer advertisements and other informational texts, including the *DSM-IV-TR*, codify symptoms in phrases like "loss of interest," which then become shibboleths for diagnosis. Framing one's

experiences in diagnostic terms becomes commonplace in a late modern society that generates discourse alongside activity and that values the speed of
communication. And yet, the consequences of diagnosis, or even of understanding the self in relation to potential diagnosis, are significant increases in
practices of uncritical self-doctoring.

These readings of the *DSM* suggest the power and necessity of a rhetorical
approach to mental health care. Fostering critical reading strategies among
individuals—attending to the historical antecedents of and to the rhetorical constructions within apparently objective documents such as the *DSM*—
potentially encourages self-care rather than self-doctoring. A healthy suspicion
of diagnostic criteria may lead some individuals to more complex understandings of their experiences: while they may make use of treatments, they may also
modify their acceptance of an illness identity that only partially defines them.
Not only might such pedagogical strategies enable the tactical use of diagnostic
terminology to achieve therapies that are meaningful to individuals, but they
might also acknowledge the cultural location of mental illness itself. Such
an acknowledgment could lead individuals to understand their experiences not
merely as symptoms but as embedded responses to complex social scenes.
In response, individuals might come to rely on *multiple* discourses for therapeutic interventions rather than simply on those of biological psychiatry

Self-Monitoring, Self-Modeling, and
the Persuasive Power of Depression

If depression becomes available through subjective reporting and self-
surveillance, it serves as an important indicator of contemporary attitudes
toward the self and practices of self-doctoring. Scholars from a variety of disciplines have commented on the intimate connection between depression and
the self, calling depression "an illness of the self"[34] and a disorder "of self and
self-identity."[35] This connection extends not just to those who suffer from
depression, but to everyone whose contact with the illness serves as an empathetic communion and a fundamentally human experience. According to
Stanley Jackson, "someone else's depression . . . is ultimately going to come
home to us as a fellow human being who also has needs, who also knows something about personal losses, disappointments, and failures, who also knows
something about being sad and dejected, and who has some capacity for distressed response to such a distressing state. With such distress, we are at the
very heart of being human."[36] Indeed, the assumed humanity of depression
serves to confuse its definition, according to David Karp, "unlike most illnesses
that we either do or do not have, everyone feels 'depressed' periodically."[37] Both
Jackson and Karp seem to conflate an emotional state with illness: in common
speech, the word *depression* itself applies equally to mild and passing sadness as

it does to mental illness. Such lexical imprecision encourages healthy identities that nevertheless encompass a certain level of illness. We even take pride in the knowledge that has come from our own losses, disappointments, and failures. When the self automatically contains potential illness, it becomes the target for additional surveillance. In an NIMH pamphlet describing depression in women, readers are told that people with dysthymia, a milder but more chronic form of depression, "are frequently lacking in zest and enthusiasm for life, living a joyless and fatigued existence that seems almost a natural outgrowth of their personalities."[38] In this statement, women's personalities are already suspect; in fact, they may not be distinguishable from illness. As a consequence of such statements, the gendered self requires extensive monitoring for signs that could suggest a need for medical intervention.

Beyond recognizing the tragedy of being human within the face of depression, recent pharmacological advances have led to surprising questions about the coherence of the self. In *Listening to Prozac*, Peter Kramer introduced the potential for psychopharmacology to produce profound changes in self-perception. After the conclusion of her treatment with Prozac, one of Kramer's patients, Tess, reports the return of some of her symptoms by saying "I am not myself."[39] Kramer describes his interaction with her:

> When I asked her to expand on what she meant, Tess said she no longer felt like herself when certain aspects of her ailment—lack of confidence, feelings of vulnerability—returned, even to a small degree. . . . Suddenly those intimate and consistent traits are not-me, they are alien, they are defect, they are illness. . . . Tess had come to understand herself—the person she had been for so many years—to be mildly ill. . . . Prozac redefined Tess's understanding of what was essential to her and what was intrusive and pathological. [40]

Kramer's analysis, that Prozac is responsible for Tess's newfound sense of self, leads him to question the limits of a "cosmetic psychopharmacology," where undesirable personality traits might be tweaked and adjusted via medications such as Prozac. [41] Kramer's phrase, with special emphasis on his first term, *cosmetic*, has been taken up by bioethicists concerned with so-called enhancement technologies that serve social rather than strictly medical purposes. In the early Prozac days, there was a sense that the drug and others like it would give individuals ultimate control over their selves, but the drug has done less to help individuals remake themselves than it has to help them fit into prevailing social expectations. In John Hewett, Michael Fraser, and Leslie Beth Berger's analysis, for example, the potential for Prozac to "become a basis for a social identity" remains unrealized as individuals use the drug merely "to adjust their mood to cultural requirements rather than to experiment with the possibilities of the self."[42] Rather than signaling the creation of a new, more malleable self,

Prozac seems to have encouraged a more conservative, conforming self; it has produced practices of self-doctoring.

More than a decade after *Listening to Prozac*, Kramer recounts the phenomenon with which that text was concerned: his patients experienced a change from being "[t]empermentally cautious and pessimistic" to achieving "assertiveness and optimism."[43] Describing the latter qualities as a "self-assured state," Kramer points out that his patients adjusted their *temperaments* to achieve more socially acceptable, confident *selves*. Thus, within the discourse of depression (and additionally within the discourse of Prozac), selves are vulnerable to the social reception of their temperaments, personalities, and emotions. Each of these features, the discourse maintains, can be positively adjusted through medication, and the failure to do so risks further alienation. The self, manipulated though various therapies, even purchased through the ingestion of medications, achieves socially acceptable qualities such as assertiveness or optimism. This commodification of the self results in what Justine Coupland and Richard Gwyn term a "body project" aimed at producing "preferred and fashionably desirable versions of outward form."[44] In the case of depression, the body project encompasses practices of self-doctoring, practices that encourage individuals both to serve as their own doctors and to present identities that conform to the gendered representations of health.

These practices of self-doctoring are, at least in part, motivated by what Kenneth Gergen calls a "vocabulary of deficit," which originates within mental health professionals' attempts to explain undesirable behavior. Accepting these explanations, however, individuals come to judge themselves and their peers through this negative vocabulary. [45] The NIMH brochure's description of dysthymic people as "lacking in zest and enthusiasm for life" is not simply a *description* of individuals suffering from an illness; it is also a *prescription* for all individuals to value "zest" and "enthusiasm" and to take measures to achieve these qualities. Such a vocabulary of deficit contributes to the visibility of illness identities, and particularly the visibility of the gendered expectations of the self. Within the discourse of depression, an emphasis on surveillance, on producing a recognizable identity, encourages self-doctoring, particularly of affective experiences and displays.

Especially for women, who have historically been targeted by social advice, regulation and observation, the self is vulnerable to discursive (and pharmaceutical) regulation.[46] In a qualitative study of eleven women suffering from depression, Dana Crowley Jack explains that the women "describe their depression as precipitated . . . by the recognition that they have lost *themselves* in trying to establish an intimacy that was never attained."[47] Jack explains that both the attempts at intimacy and the loss of self are rhetorical gestures (though she does not use this terminology): the women find themselves no longer the subjects of their own lives, and this is displayed in the rhetorical

choices they make in their therapy sessions. The discursive loss of agency parallels the psychological loss, suggesting that women are literally silencing their
selves, to borrow Jack's title. But whether and how the self speaks—through a
vocabulary of deficit, with the aid of pharmaceutical interventions, or not at
all—is largely a product of the discourse of depression, which shapes the audible statements and visible representations of health and illness through which
the self is experienced.

Depression's Apparent Gender

As opposed to biological sex, gender is a social category that takes shape only
within cultural and historical scenes. In the World Health Organization's words,
gender refers to "the socially constructed roles, behaviour, activities and attributes that a particular society considers appropriate for men and women."[48]
Further, distinct gender roles "may give rise to gender inequalities, i.e. differences between men and women that systematically favour one group. In turn,
such inequalities can lead to inequities between men and women in both
health status and access to health care."[49] The consequences of gender are
material as well as social: roles and behaviors deemed appropriate for one
group may predispose them to illness, because they are economically or socially
distanced from quality care, because their activities put them in hazardous
environments, or even because they are *assumed* to be vulnerable. In the case of
depression—an illness regularly described as affecting women at twice the rate
as men[50]—this has significant consequences for *both* men and women. While
cultural assumptions might result in the overdiagnosis of women and the
underdiagnosis of men with depression, they can also lead to significantly gendered understandings of health and illness more generally. If women are
assumed to be at greater risk of depression, their emotional lives become targets for additional scrutiny and surveillance, an outcome that is produced in
part through the texts that are written to ensure better mental health.
Throughout the discourse of depression, gender becomes a central category
around which practices of self-doctoring develop, and it in turn becomes a significant product of these practices.

Similar to the definition of *discourse* as a regulatory mechanism that is constantly reenacted via the statements that constitute it, this definition of *gender*
implies both representation, the *display* of stereotypical gender roles, and construction, the *shaping* of particular forms of masculinity and femininity, of subjectivities. Cultural anxieties about gender play out on the stage of illnesses
such as depression, and thus the articulations of those illnesses reflect back on
the ideas and performances of gender. Associating women's emotions with
potential depression, for example, both makes women more vulnerable to
illness and reiterates cultural stereotypes about women's so-called normal

emotional lives. Within the discourse of depression, the *self* becomes subject to a series of monitoring and doctoring practices in part because of the imprecise definition of the illness. Women, particularly white, middle-class women, who read and accept messages about their affective lives, are especially vulnerable to the circulating messages about mental health and illness. For women of color, such messages are often only tangentially inclusive, affording them even fewer options for self-definition. These circumstances reflect the content and quality of statements directed at women and also the prevailing understanding of depression as primarily a middle-class (white) woman's illness.[51]

Meri Nana-Ama Danquah comments in her memoir on black women's lack of rhetorical options for discussing depression. She writes: "Sadly, it is not only white people who are unable to see beyond the ornamentation that is placed on black women's lives. I have had conversations about my depression with black people—both men and women—that were similar. . . . When there aren't dismissive questions, patronizing statements, or ludicrous suggestions, there is silence. As if there are no acceptable ways, no appropriate words to begin a dialogue about this illness."[52] This silence is repeated throughout the public discourse of depression: very few articles in my corpus mention the race (or class) of the individuals whose lives illuminate depression for readers. In over two hundred articles, only six use the descriptor *black* and only five use *white* to describe the ethnicity of individuals or groups of people. Articles with titles such as "Quiet Demons in Black Life" further emphasize the silence surrounding depression in nonwhite communities.[53] Similarly, indications of class are notably absent from the corpus, with the exception of articles in the *New York Times* series entitled "The Neediest Cases," which describe the lives of individuals who have benefited from the *New York Times* charitable fund. The prototypical depressed woman, meant to stand in for all women (and, potentially, all men as well), serves as an icon in the discourse that oversimplifies identity, just as the biochemical explanation for her illness oversimplifies etiology. Both mask more complex realities and experiences; both would benefit from more sustained critical analysis.

The discourse of depression constructs a gendered self subject to illness through a variety of rhetorical gestures, one of the most powerful of which is the use of statistics. In fact, one of the most consistent pieces of knowledge that circulates within the discourse of depression is the finding that women are approximately twice as likely to be depressed as men.[54] According to NIMH, each year 12 percent of U.S. women and 6.6 percent of U.S. men are affected by a depressive disorder.[55] According to the World Health Organization, "depression is women's leading cause of disease burden" when measured in disability-adjusted life years.[56] The consistency of this finding across a variety of age ranges and cultures has become so much a part of our understanding of the illness that simply being female puts one at risk for depression. For example, *Diagnosis According to the DSM-IV*, an instructional film for mental health professionals, documents ten patient interviews as examples of illness. A panel of experts discusses each interview extensively. In the film, Barbara (a middle-aged, white woman) represents the diagnosis of Major Depressive Disorder (MDD). Clearly, the choice of a female patient is meant to reflect the greater number of women who apparently suffer from clinical depression. However, the choice of Barbara also helps to reinforce assumptions about who is susceptible to the disorder. In the discussion that follows Barbara's interview, the sense of depression as a "woman's disease" is introduced by Steven Moldin, a clinical psychologist. Near the beginning of the discussion, he points out that "Barbara is very typical as a sufferer of major depression given the fact that she is a woman." Moldin follows this remark with a listing of statistics demonstrating the gender gap in depression; he does not elaborate on any other way that Barbara might be considered "very typical" of depressed patients (and neither do any of the other panelists). In fact, the conversation turns immediately to Barbara's atypical ability to articulate her symptoms. This discussion, staged to help clinicians use the diagnostic criteria of the *DSM-IV*, does not question or even qualify the equation: depressed patient = woman.[57]

Beyond the clinical scene of diagnosis and the broader cultural imagination, researchers on depression also seem prone to adopting this same equation. In a broad review of the scholarship on gender and depression, Susan Nolen-Hoeksema uses data from "studies of people who were depressed enough to seek treatment, and studies in which cut-off scores from depression questionnaires were used to define depression" to argue that "no matter how you define depression, after puberty women show more depression than men."[58] Her conclusion is based on two rhetorically complicated phenomena: the studies assess individuals who understand themselves to be sick and individuals who respond to a written questionnaire. Both standards are subject to the discourse of depression. The individuals in the first set of studies had to understand themselves as depressed and be willing to seek treatment, and, as Nolen-Hoeksema admits, women are more likely than men to visit mental health professionals.[59] The individuals in the second set of studies interacted directly with texts that asked questions about affective experiences, and such questions are inevitably shaped by prevailing articulations of the illness. In both cases, the studies are likely to reveal exactly what Nolen-Hoeksema reports: women are more likely to *appear* depressed than men. While this may be considered an established scientific fact, it has also taken on the guise of a self-fulfilling prophecy.

Early feminist criticism of mental health categories suggest that women's "madness" is more appropriately explained as a healthy response to social and physical oppression.[60] As recently as 1992, Ellen McGrath, a prominent clinical psychologist and member of the APA's National Taskforce on Women and

Depression, published *When Feeling Bad Is Good*, an "innovative self-help program" that distinguishes between two distinct depressions. For McGrath, "Healthy Depression" provides the impetus for change and self-evaluation, while "Unhealthy Depression" is a debilitating illness. Appearing at the beginning of a decade of increased pharmaceutical intervention into our moods, McGrath's text works to delineate the boundaries of appropriate medical interventions, but it also reminds us that there are good reasons that women may be depressed.[61] While such feminist criticism has pointed out social inequities, it has done very little to disassociate women from depression. Women are still encouraged to fulfill stereotypical gender roles and they are disproportionately targeted with messages about their emotional states, which are often pictured as equivalent to illnesses.

Even texts that display surface-level gender neutrality correlate women's social and familial roles with their potential vulnerability to depression. In Kramer's *Against Depression*, the statement that "depressives are bad parents" seems to implicate both mother and father, yet in context, this judgment applies nearly exclusively to *mothers*. He writes, "What of postpartum psychosis, where a mother kills her newborns? What of suicide? What of dense anhedonia, in which a mother neglects her young children? . . . Depressives make bad parents. But the truth holds only for the intervals when the illness is active; many women who are moody during courtship will make fine wives and mothers."[62] Each of Kramer's rhetorical questions targets women, both individually and as a group.[63] Kramer's pronouncement—that depressives make bad parents, by which he means bad *mothers*—not only serves to gender depression, but also to enhance suspicion of *all* women who, though "moody during courtship" might either become "fine wives and mothers" or "kill [their] newborns." In another similar passage, Kramer discusses the undesirability of aligning oneself romantically with a depressed person. He writes: "No one wants to marry into depression. In fact, parents might (and do) advise against it: 'She's very sweet, but she strikes your father as depressive.'"[64] Here again, the general assertion turns out to be gendered, even to the extent that the father has concerns, but the mother serves as the mouthpiece for them. *Parents*, it turns out, translates to *mothers*—depressives are, in these passages, *bad mothers* and *bad wives*, not simply bad parents.[65] These examples display the consistency and subtlety of the gendering of depression, and, further, the means through which the discourse of depression constructs women in general as potentially dangerous or otherwise undesirable, both of which entail additional self-doctoring on the part of women to ameliorate.

Men do not escape the discourse of depression, and the stereotypes of strong, silent men are just as pervasive as those of dangerous, moody women. In fact, men are represented as reluctant to admit their feelings of depression, indicating their own self-silencing behaviors (however, men's depression is not described as intrinsic to their *selves* in the way that it is for women). In 2003, the NIMH launched a campaign aimed at encouraging men to seek treatment for their depression. It used the headline: "Real Men. Real Depression." Using phrases such as "It takes courage to ask for help," this campaign attempts to destigmatize depression in men, but it continues to suggest that the central illness features, "feelings of sadness, worthlessness, and excessive guilt," are associated primarily with women. Men, the pamphlet suggests, are more likely to experience "fatigue, irritability, loss of interest in work or hobbies, and sleep disturbances." Thus, male depression is more often represented as a physical rather than an emotional experience, and men are characterized as "reporting" symptoms rather than "having feelings." Within this syntax, gender is articulated along stereotypical lines and illness is read more consistently into the identities of women. Nevertheless, men's identities are also shaped through the discourse, in particular through the appropriate responses to illness represented.

The messages women and men receive through texts about depression include more than medical advice. In fact, such texts reinforce women's greater vulnerability to the illness largely by reiterating a cultural stereotype that women are "more emotional" than men. For example, a simple comparison of the first sentences of two NIMH depression pamphlets reveals this discursive construction of women's emotionality. A general-audience pamphlet begins with: "In any given 1-year period, 9.5 percent of the population, or about 18.8 million American adults, suffer from a depressive illness. The economic cost for this disorder is high, but the cost in human suffering cannot be estimated."[66] By contrast, a pamphlet directed specifically at women begins: "Life is full of emotional ups and downs. But when the 'down' times are long lasting or interfere with your ability to function, you may be suffering from a common, serious illness—depression."[67] In the general pamphlet, objective-sounding information delineates costs of the illness—a rhetorical choice that values productive labor (or its loss in economic terms) and that gestures toward "human suffering" without quantifying it. Instead of such objectivity, the women's pamphlet starts immediately with emotional language, personalizing its address by using the second-person: "You may be suffering." This serves not only to invite the reader to view herself as possibly depressed, but also to reinforce the idea that women's lives are naturally and inevitably filled with changing emotions. Texts about depression encourage constant practices of self-doctoring in order to help women avoid the always potential transformation of emotion into illness. Gender is thus deeply embedded in the discourse of depression.

At the turn of the twenty-first century, depression is a fundamentally rhetorical phenomenon. In addition to its material existence, the illness occasions a powerful discourse that shapes individual, gendered health and illness identities. Talk and personal storytelling, often aimed at accounting for particular pharmaceutical interventions, proliferates around the illness. Diagnostic rubrics organize the collection of symptoms and encourage self- and other-reporting practices that further embed the illness in language. And, the illness itself stands as a negative model, a dangerous result of allowing the self to eschew acceptable models for gendered and healthy behavior. Responding to these rhetorical pressures, practices of self-doctoring, even self-diagnosis, promise to safeguard individuals and to hold illness at bay. Yet these practices become ever more restricted as they focus attention toward biochemical malfunctions rather than acknowledging the rhetorical embedding of all experiences of health and illness. Such an acknowledgment might, however, result in forms of self-care that offer more satisfactory health and illness identities. If individuals take time to examine the messages they receive about their own health and illness, they may come to recognize patterns that constellate around particular illnesses such as depression. In so doing, they may also come to begin a multivoiced dialogue about these patterns, opening up discursive possibilities rather than accepting narrow biochemical responses to their experiences.

2

Articulate Depression

The Discursive Legacy of Biological Psychiatry

Understanding depression as a rhetorical phenomenon opens a space for analysis that attends to the discursive forms that shape the illness and the identities of its sufferers. The signs of illness—withdrawal from social contact, recurrent painful and guilty thoughts, loss of enjoyment in activities and interactions—paint sufferers as profoundly silenced, yet the volume of contemporary talk and text belies this characterization. The discourse of depression articulates the illness within a series of gendered identities in both senses of that verb: *joining* features into a single illness, and *pronouncing* distinctly the identities associated with it. Historically, this verb also encompassed the activities of coming to terms, via the acceptance of articles or conditions, and of capitulating to such terms.[1] These now obsolete definitions nevertheless echo within the self-doctoring practices mandated within the contemporary discourse of depression. As individuals define themselves using the vocabulary common to medical practice, they relinquish personal autonomy in favor of medical recognition and pharmaceutical treatment. While such capitulations may result in effective treatments for some, evidence suggests that for a significant number of individuals these interventions are of limited value. A rhetorical analysis, then, makes visible the joints by which the illness itself is assembled and voiced.

Direct-to-consumer advertisements represent the most obvious textual site for locating practices of self-doctoring, as they encourage individuals to act as their own physicians and to model their behaviors and self-assessments on the "ideal" images projected. According to the U.S. Government Accountability Office, spending on direct-to-consumer marketing materials for pharmaceuticals nearly tripled between 1997 and 2005, from $1.1 billion to $4.2 billion annually.[2] This increase attests to a business model that has moved prescription drug promotion out of the doctor's office and into homes via television and print media. It also represents a shift within medical rhetoric, which has traditionally consisted of doctor-patient dyads and a relatively closed system of expert knowledge. In the late twentieth century, however, the rapid growth of direct-to-consumer pharmaceutical promotion and the development of information delivery systems such as WebMD have reconfigured the system of expertise and the balance of power in medical encounters.[3] Such developments precipitate new medical rhetorics, especially those configured around the authority of pharmaceutical companies. Among the most highly marketed pharmaceuticals are the class of antidepressants known as the selective serotonin reuptake inhibitors (SSRIs, such as Prozac, Paxil, and Zoloft), and their cousins the selective serotonin norepinephrine reuptake inhibitors (SSNRIs, such as Cymbalta and Effexor), which additionally block the reuptake of norepinephrine. These drugs have likely saved and improved many lives, but they have also undoubtedly *changed* what it means to be alive and mentally well (or ill).[4] These new definitions of mental health result not directly from the new chemical compounds and their effects on temperament or brain functioning, but from the rhetoric that attends their development, marketing, and use. Depression and the drugs used to treat it have entered the public lexicon thoroughly and irrevocably. Prozac, and the pharmaceutical complex it metonymically represents, is now a resource for constructing individual and collective understandings of the self and its mental health needs.[5]

The successes of the pharmaceutical industry have conditioned the statements it is possible to make about depression and the self. Such statements are not mere rhetoric, but rather consequential heuristics through which individuals experience their lives and their selves. In one of my interviews with women experiencing symptoms of depression, Stephanie admitted, "I honestly do think that I have a chemical imbalance" even as she adamantly refused to accept medical or other therapeutic interventions in her life. While Stephanie has not fully embraced the illness identity that requires pharmaceutical intervention, she is clearly beginning to see herself in biochemical terms. For medical rhetoricians, understanding the linguistic impact of biological psychiatry offers a chance to explore how *individuals* such as Stephanie become *patients* and how *illnesses* become *identities*. Language filters and organizes experience, naming and categorizing both feelings and symptoms as "normal" or "dysfunctional." Alongside the scientific developments of biological psychiatry, a set of standard linguistic structures encourages isolated acts of self-doctoring by encompassing broad and strategically imprecise definitions of illness, by offering figurative and narrative descriptions that model gendered responses to illnesses such as depression, and by making available genres such as the symptoms quiz that direct individuals to their doctors' offices. Therefore, in addition to critiques of the contemporary *science* of depression, we need careful rhetorical analyses of the *language* of depression. As a result of such analyses, and by participating in them, individuals may develop more complex, indeed, more *dialogical* practices of self-care.

Biological Psychiatry and a Narrowing Discursive Field

The new paradigm of biological psychiatry developed out of the context of mid-century concerns over institutionalization, problematic somatic treatments, and the beginnings of the pharmaceutical industry.[6] The third edition of the *DSM*, published in 1987, announced a dramatic shift away from psychodynamic principles and toward research-based psychiatry, bringing with it a new vocabulary of diagnostic reliability.[7] Perhaps nowhere is this so well displayed as in the cultural history of depression over the last half-century. As *Listening to Prozac* announced in 1993, the transformative effects of psychopharmaceuticals appeared to promise the obsolescence of lengthy psychotherapy to treat depression and related disorders. While the fantasy of a miracle pill has not been entirely realized, the discursive terrain has nevertheless migrated from a psychotherapeutic model, where patient talk is central to treatment, and interactions with health-care institutions are characterized by *dialogue* with multiple textual sources; to a biological model, where patient talk is largely instrumental, directed unilaterally at doctors in the service of requesting medications, and interactions with health-care institutions are characterized by a pharmaceutical-inspired *monologue*. Edward Shorter dubs this period of psychiatric history the shift "from Freud to Prozac."[8] In other words, it is the period that witnesses a change of allegiance from talk therapy to chemical intervention. The discursive quality of this shift often remains opaque, but a critical rhetorical evaluation reveals the impulse toward self-doctoring that reinforces biochemical responses to illness.[9]

The rapid growth and influence of the pharmaceutical industry and the additional attention directed at depression following the declaration that it is the leading cause of disability and the fourth leading contributor to the global burden of disease[10] require a critique of what Andrew Lakoff calls "pharmaceutical reason." Lakoff uses this term to refer to the "strategic logic" of biological psychiatry that results from the interactions of powerful health-care institutions. Missing from his list of powerful contributors to pharmaceutical reason, however, is the discourse through which institutions communicate and solidify their power.[11] A proliferation of messages about depression at the end of the twentieth century has not resulted in a diversity of approaches to the illness. Instead, in popular discourse, depression has been largely reduced to a biological phenomenon, which has left little room for competing understandings. Because language used about depression significantly shapes the illness—that is, by determining which experiences and responses qualify as depression—and the possible subject positions in relation to it, this narrowing represents a significant shift in the versions of the self that are linguistically available. A careful analysis of the language surrounding depression, therefore, offers a chance to understand better these discursive pressures and perhaps to reinstate a dialogic orientation toward mental health and illness.

In February 1998, a two-page advertisement for Eli Lilly's Prozac appeared in *Time*. The left page shows a cartoon depiction of a leafless tree against a blue background; the right page shows the tree complete with green canopy against a bright orange background (figure 2). Under the images are the phrases "Depression isolates" and "Prozac can help." In these images there is an explicit acknowledgment of the social embedding of the self: the "cured" image contains not just the tree, but an oversized cartoon bird nesting in its branches, and in the text below this image is the statement: "Chances are someone you know is blossoming again because of it [Prozac]." In a companion advertisement published in the same year, depression appears as a rain cloud against a black background, a contrast to the sunny sky under the influence of Prozac. This version of the advertisement observes that "Chances are someone you know is feeling sunny again because of it [Prozac]." Carefully gender-neutral in their symbolic representations of depression as either "seasonal" or "meteorological," these advertisements nevertheless imply a gendered subjectivity in their choice of descriptors—*blossoming* and *sunny*—for the individual who is returned to health via a prescription for Prozac. Whether the patient is imagined to be male (but perhaps not *masculine*, having been returned to "blossoming" health) or female (but perhaps not *intellectual*, having been returned to "sunny" feelings), the promise of treatment is additionally a promise of transport from an affectively flat realm of isolation into a vibrant world of social integration that validates and rewards appropriately gendered performances of the self.

This movement of the subject occurs by means of an almost alchemical exchange of a doctor's written prescription slip for a medication dispensed at a pharmacy, yet the movement of the subject beyond the limits of "depression" also implicates a social network beyond the biomedical provinces of doctor's office and drugstore. Both versions of the advertisement acknowledge a community of sufferers encompassing more than the individual reader; each states that "Prozac has been prescribed for more than 17 million Americans," and each offers a greeting—"Welcome back"—as the final tagline, a move that reverses readers' expectations of closure by inaugurating a new sociality via the pharmaceutical treatment. These texts encourage readers to understand themselves as potentially ill and in need of intervention to perform socially. In addition, they gesture toward a network of potential depression sufferers one might know, or from whom one might be isolated by depression in one's own turn.

Three years later, the social isolation in the Prozac advertisements intensifies and narrows to the singular depressed individual within advertisements for Pfizer's antidepressant, Zoloft. These texts feature a white egg- or rock-like

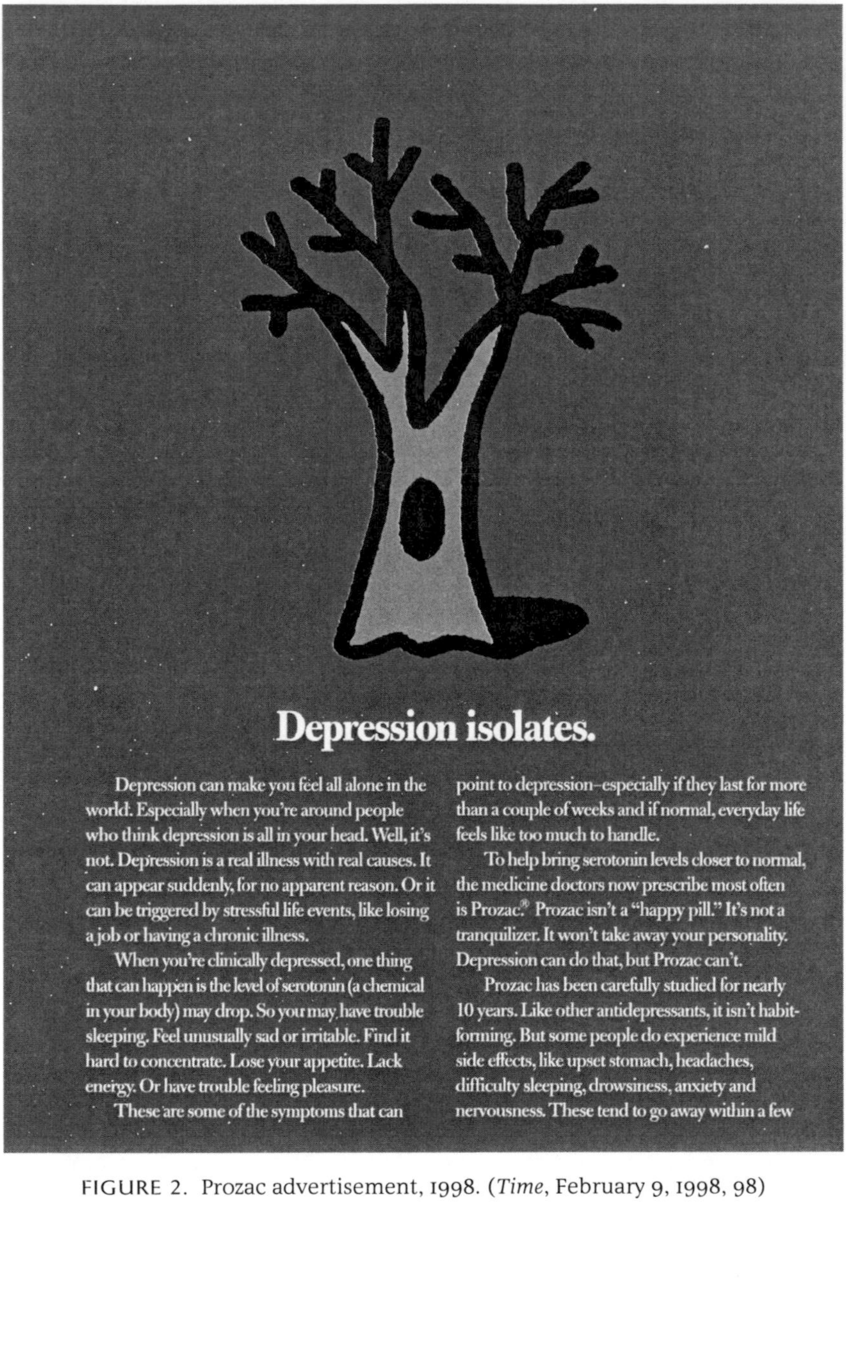

Depression isolates.

Depression can make you feel all alone in the world. Especially when you're around people who think depression is all in your head. Well, it's not. Depression is a real illness with real causes. It can appear suddenly, for no apparent reason. Or it can be triggered by stressful life events, like losing a job or having a chronic illness.

When you're clinically depressed, one thing that can happen is the level of serotonin (a chemical in your body) may drop. So you may have trouble sleeping. Feel unusually sad or irritable. Find it hard to concentrate. Lose your appetite. Lack energy. Or have trouble feeling pleasure.

These are some of the symptoms that can point to depression–especially if they last for more than a couple of weeks and if normal, everyday life feels like too much to handle.

To help bring serotonin levels closer to normal, the medicine doctors now prescribe most often is Prozac.® Prozac isn't a "happy pill." It's not a tranquilizer. It won't take away your personality. Depression can do that, but Prozac can't.

Prozac has been carefully studied for nearly 10 years. Like other antidepressants, it isn't habit-forming. But some people do experience mild side effects, like upset stomach, headaches, difficulty sleeping, drowsiness, anxiety and nervousness. These tend to go away within a few

FIGURE 2. Prozac advertisement, 1998. (*Time*, February 9, 1998, 98)

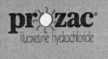

Prozac can help.

weeks of starting treatment, and usually aren't serious enough to make most people stop taking it. However, if you are concerned about a side effect, or if you develop a rash, tell your doctor right away. And don't forget to tell your doctor about any other medicines you are taking. Some people should not take Prozac, especially people on MAO inhibitors.

As you start feeling better, your doctor can suggest therapy or other means to help you work through your depression. Remember, Prozac is a prescription medicine, and it isn't right for everyone. Only your doctor can decide if Prozac is right for you–or for someone you love.

Prozac has been prescribed for more than 17 million Americans. Chances are someone you know is blossoming again because of it.

prozac
fluoxetine hydrochloride

Welcome back.

Please see important information on following page. *Lilly*
http://www.lilly.com

FIGURE 2. (*continued*)

creature against a solid black background. The creature expresses illness (and health) within simplistic emotional iconography: it cries, frowns, and sighs when ill; it smiles and bounces when cured. In one print version of the advertisement, the creature sits crying under the overhang of a cliff; in another, it cries under a crescent moon (figure 3). In both, the darkness of night aligns symbolically with the settings imagined by the Prozac advertisements: the sparse foliage of winter and the flat gray weather of a rainstorm. But the black night is more intensely isolating, unrelieved as it is by any hint of color or a return to the dawn of health. Again, the Zoloft advertisements are carefully gender-neutral, though the shape, the moon, and the tears imply a feminized, if not necessarily female, subject. In the years since this campaign began, the creature has appeared in several guises on the Zoloft Web site, including one image where it is pushing a shopping cart and appears to be wearing lipstick, and another that includes two creatures sharing a meal, one of whom again appears to be wearing lipstick. This character, then, represents the depressed individual as primarily featureless—indeed without arms, legs, or a body—but marks her, nevertheless, as displaying her gender appropriately when she has been returned to social functioning via Zoloft.

In the black-and-white print advertisements, the depressed individual is isolated not simply by the setting but by the text, which begins with a series of second-person declarative statements: "You know when you're not feeling like yourself. You're tired all the time. . . . You know when you just don't feel right." These statements direct attention inward, away from social interaction. The reader is isolated in self-knowledge and is not invited to imagine or recognize *others* as similarly afflicted. In the middle of the text, a "dramatization" offers an explanation for depression that internalizes the illness and further distances it from a community of sufferers. In the first line drawing, a neurotransmitter with very few serotonin bubbles circulating receives the label "chemical imbalance" in the second, the neurotransmitter with "reuptake" blockers in place is crowded with serotonin bubbles and receives the label "with Zoloft." This graphic representation encourages readers to see the illness as a microscopic internal malfunction; it isolates the cause of depression just as the larger context of the advertisement has isolated the depressed individual. The tagline for this campaign—"When you know more about what's wrong, you can help make it right.™"—involves the individual in his or her recovery to the extent that he or she takes up the advertisement's explanation as self-knowledge. Making it right—increasing the available serotonin bubbles—links knowledge, particularly self-knowledge, to pharmaceutical action. Indeed, the burden of diagnosis appears to have shifted further toward the individual, who is commanded to "*Talk* to your doctor . . . *Call* 1–800–6–ZOLOFT or *visit* www.ZOLOFT.com" (emphasis added)—all verbal steps the subject can take, but also *monological* steps that encourage self-diagnosis.

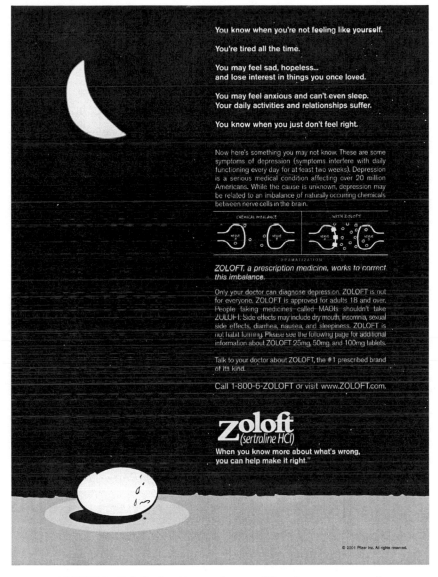

FIGURE 3. Zoloft advertisement, 2001. (*Time*, June 4, 2001, n.p)

Beginning in 2006, Eli Lilly created a campaign for its new antidepressant, Cymbalta, using human actors in a series of tableaus that translate depression into a hypersocial setting. In television and print ads, as well as on a Web site dedicated to the drug, the scenes accompany a series of questions about the effects of depression. The key question, "Who does depression hurt?" is answered with a universalizing "Everyone," and with images of children, spouses, and even the family dog, who sits patiently by the door, unwalked. The correlative question, "Where does depression hurt?" is answered with the similarly universalizing "Everywhere," and by successive images of individuals holding their heads or remaining in bed. The campaign, which includes a "DepressionHurts" Web site, prominently features a depressed mother who turns her back on her children's tea party. The accompanying text points out that "many of [her] relationships" are endangered by depression. Not only does this image cite the "bad mother" trope common in texts about depression, but it also reads women's relationships as primarily domestic and nurturing rather than as professional or as occurring among peers. The tagline accompanying this campaign is a statement of individual empowerment: "Depression hurts, but you don't have to." The "healthy" scenes of social interaction, often in a kitchen or involving food, reflect an effort to include male actors—though they are far outnumbered by female actors—and suggest that "everyone" is potentially subject to the illness. Nevertheless, the domestic settings and the emphasis on family cohesion imply caretaking activities, both of which are usually associated with women's roles.

Taking up the ethos of self-empowerment, these advertisements echo those for Zoloft and encourage viewers to control their own illness and health experiences, but the Cymbalta advertisements add a stronger sense of culpability for individuals who fail to seek pharmaceutical intervention. The rhetoric of the ads recasts the isolation of depression as directly harming the social world in which the individual is supposed to participate. Not just *depression* hurts "everyone," the ad implies; *you* hurt those around you when you suffer from depression. Readers of the Cymbalta ads appear already as having adopted a proactive stance toward their health-care decisions—something that the earlier Prozac and Zoloft advertisements encouraged in their rhetoric—but they now also find themselves within an expert system that resembles the paternalistic doctor-patient dyad that characterized medical encounters until the late twentieth century. Yet an important substitution has been made to this dyad: the doctor's expertise and authority has been replaced by those of the pharmaceutical company, which promises that "you don't have to" hurt (yourself and others) anymore. The benevolence of this advice masks the implied critique, namely, that an individual's failure to seek (or, more precisely, to *consume*) treatment should be read as a careless and selfish act *against* his or her social network.

The idea of the self and its responsibility for its own and others' care shifts in significant ways across these texts. In early antidepressant advertising, the self is comparable to other selves, who may also be struggling with the isolation and pain of depression. The Prozac advertisements acknowledge a chemical etiology for depression, but pose it as *a correlative or even an effect* of suffering, and couch it in tentative language: "When you're depressed, one thing that can happen is that the level of serotonin (a chemical in your brain) may drop." By the turn of the twenty-first century, the texts target this chemical model far more explicitly, so that the Zoloft advertisement includes its two-pane graphic as a simplified *explanation* for the illness, and the Cymbalta Web site offers an interactive "Science of Depression" tool that animates the apparent effects of neurotransmitters, suggesting chemical *causality*. In these later advertisements, the self has been isolated from others, and the origin of this isolation has been located with a faulty system of chemical exchange in the brain. When, in 2006, the self returns to social interaction, it does so with a far more directive message: defining depression as the product of faulty brain chemistry means that suffering from depression can no longer appear simply as a matter of the isolated self in misery; because the underlying cause can (apparently) be repaired through a simple pharmaceutical intervention, suffering depression is also an imposition upon others that the self has a moral obligation to rectify. Across these advertisements, the individual's connection to a social network diminishes as a consequence of suffering, and it returns only as a by-product of the self's responsible steps to secure medication. Consequently, where once social interaction was threatened by illness, now it is a casualty of individuals' potential refusal of pharmaceutical intervention as ultimate cure. Adoption of a medicalized view of the self and its experiences promises to reconnect the individual to community. The dynamic emerging from these advertisements marks just one recent innovation in the discourse of depression—the collective series of contemporary statements and beliefs about the illness, primary among which is the individual obligation to seek treatment—that fundamentally shapes not only our experiences of the illness, but also our experience of our*selves.*

DESPITE ADVICE to *talk* to our doctors, faith in technological solutions seems at this historical moment to override attention to language. The "biological turn" in psychiatry appears dominant, supplanting earlier talk therapies, which relied on communicative rather than physiological interactions. Heralding this new biological psychiatry—a process achieved in part through the publication of the phrase and its semantic equivalents—has not, however, displaced the need for rhetorical supplements, but it has established a desire for the "quick fix" of medication (and the cost-effectiveness of lists of drugs approved for insurance reimbursement). This desire leads many—including prominent psychiatrists and medical specialists—to imagine a future cure for depression that takes human language out of the equation.

One such apparently utopian future is promised by advances in pharmacogenomics, a field that combines genetic and pharmaceutical research, according to Dr. Richard Friedman, writing in the *New York Times* in June 2007. Friedman predicts that "it will soon be possible for a psychiatrist to biologically personalize treatments. With a simple blood test, the doctor will be able to characterize a patient's unique genetic profile, determining what biological type of depression the patient has and which antidepressant is likely to work best." Friedman views these advances as enabling more "personal" treatment, because they will help doctors make choices that reflect scientific assumptions about genetic predispositions. "Soon," he writes, "your psychiatrist will really get to know you—not just your mind, but your brain, too." The assumption here is that the *personal* and the *genetic* are synonymous and that a thorough knowledge of a patient's genetic makeup provides the most significant form of understanding between doctor and patient. According to Friedman, technology will cut out the intermediary direct-to-consumer advertisements because patients will no longer be persuaded by generalizations; they will listen to their genes—which will speak, through their blood, directly to their doctors—instead of to their pharmaceuticals. The intimacy promised in Friedman's future doctor-patient interaction ironically requires very little social interaction, but—as direct-to-consumer advertising points up—depression is nothing if not a social, and consequently personal, complex. Friedman's utopian technology, threatened by these social and rhetorical realities of the illness it is intended to cure, seeks to suppress the ambiguities of discourse, to cut out language, and thereby to reduce depression from illness to disease.

A similar desire to distance depression from the language that expresses it pervades Peter Kramer's polemic *Against Depression*. His primary claim—that we do not take depression seriously as a disease—certainly resonates with the discursive construction of depression as a relationship between the expectations and lived experiences of the self. Indeed, Kramer usefully articulates the argument that depression has been constructed as both *more* and *less* than an illness. He writes, "Depression is more than an illness—it has a sacred aspect," referring to the belief that depression can provide insight, reveal profound truths, inspire great accomplishments. But, "depression is [also] less than an illness," as when it is seen as "a heavy dose of the artistic temperament, so that the symptoms of depression are merely personality traits."[12] Kramer sees these conflicting understandings not as the product of a powerful discourse of depression, however, but as the result of too weak a faith in technology. Kramer proposes to solve the dilemma of an illness that is also not one by shoring up our faith in a medical model that, offering a definitive cure, would apparently render language irrelevant.

In his desire to separate the medical phenomenon of depression from its discursive setting, Kramer points to significant problems in contemporary articulations of health and illness.[13] He tells of a colleague's decision to leave a patient's depression untreated "in the service of a process of self-exploration."[14] Noting that this would once have seemed unremarkable to him, Kramer now questions such choices: "Is there another disease with which a doctor would make this choice? If a patient had cancer or diabetes and seemed psychologically the better for it—humbled, taken down a notch—still, we would treat the condition vigorously."[15] For Kramer, the colleague's choice has become incomprehensible within the new disease discourse Kramer himself has adopted. Kramer's colleague, however, is operating within a competing popular discourse, which constructs depression as an opportunity for self-discovery. To remove illness from discourse and treat it objectively and arhetorically holds the appeal of remedying the inhumanities of which disease discourse is capable, but it is ultimately an impossible move. We do not operate outside of discourse, and so we cannot be so naïve as to think that we can sequester illness away from its discursive habitat or that a "medical model" is somehow free of the influence of rhetoric.

Indeed, Kramer lapses into the popular discourse of depression even as he argues for avoiding such deviations from "objectivity." He makes apparently casual statements that, rather than reinforcing his "objective" disease discourse, recirculate the notions of depression that ties the illness to lived emotions. "I became immersed in depression," he writes. "Not my own. I was in my forties and contented enough in the slog through midlife."[16] Characterizing midlife as a "slog," Kramer voices a cultural commonplace about the difficulties of aging, employing the metaphor of a slow and painful journey. His phrasing also sets up a false equation between mood and illness. Kramer was not depressed; he was "contented enough." Thus, had he been depressed, he would *not* have been content. Depression is opposed to contentment, rather than to physical health (the opposite of *disease*). Treating depression as categorically different from ordinary sadness and the routine annoyances and tragedies of life turns out to be difficult even for a medical professional who has dedicated himself to precisely this task. Kramer is not alone: in his study and memoir, Lewis Wolpert reports that "the two terms most closely linked to depression were grief and sadness."[17] The illness is inseparable from potentially "normal" affective states, and it is continually reconstructed that way in each textual and verbal repetition. This is the power of the discourse of depression: it binds the illness to moods and common affective experiences, ensuring that the boundaries of health are never entirely clear.

It has become commonplace for writers on depression to describe it as an illness that confounds communication. For instance, Nell Casey writes of the "desiccated language that is now the core of discussions of despair" in the introduction to her collection of writers' essays about their own depressions.[18] Nevertheless, the inadequacies of language ensure a constant generation of further words; the present failures of language guarantee future utterances. In this way, the discourse of depression realizes the illness as a site of constant textual production. Further, the words we use to describe depression and its treatments, outcomes, and cultural meanings—even the apparently inarticulate ones—construct the indistinct boundaries and gendered identities attached to the illness. Words succeed, but they do not provide the definitive communication of the experience of depression. Instead, words construct and maintain the sometimes conflicting understandings of depression that we hold; they show us how to be depressed and how to be healthy. The words in direct-to-consumer advertisements provide a condensed visual and textual argument for the existence of depression and for the gendered illness identities it constellates.

Constructing Illness Identities: Direct-to-Consumer Advertisements and the Verbal-Visual Rhetoric of Depression

The woman at the center of the photograph is the only one in focus; we recognize the crowd around her as people, but they are devoid of identifying features other than the shape of a hat or the dark impression of a necktie (figure 4). White, block-lettered words surround the woman: *fatigue, sleep problems, worry, restlessness, muscle tension, irritability, anxiety.* This direct-to-consumer advertisement for the antianxiety and antidepressant medication Paxil, produced and marketed by Glaxo-SmithKline, provides a visual representation of the textual landscape of mental health and illness in the United States.[19] Words saturate the image, graphically and rhetorically bounding the woman. Words name the physical and affective experiences that constitute her state of "chronic anxiety." Indeed, in this advertisement, mental illness fundamentally becomes visible as a relationship between key words and the individuals that they either bring into focus or obscure.

In a similar direct-to-consumer advertisement for the "controlled release" once-a-day formulation of PaxilCR, another woman is isolated, this time by a vertical barrier of printed words: *Depressed Mood, Loss of Interest, Sleep Problems, Difficulty Concentrating, Agitation, Restlessness* (figure 5). Across this barrier, a man and a boy look solemnly, almost accusingly at her, while she fails to return their gaze. The words seem to intervene in whatever relationship they might have, claiming center stage for the "depression" that pushes the human actors into the wings. In each of these advertisements, words translate experiences into symptoms; words isolate the women from social clarity and connection; and words label individuals with the medical conditions "chronic anxiety" and "depression." In these advertisements, words and images combine to display an illness identity that is gendered, mute except for its definitional keywords, and isolated. It is an identity crystallized from the discourse of depression and powerfully persuasive of practices of self-doctoring.

Taking these two advertisements as representative of the larger discourse of depression, the first complication surfaces as a definitional one: if Paxil treats both anxiety and depression, what connects and differentiates these two illnesses? An assumed common cause—a chemical imbalance—links these two illnesses and justifies the application of the same cure to each. In addition, similar manifestations—the two illnesses share some of the same expressions of symptoms—also link anxiety and depression. In the advertisements, these connections are represented by the women "patients" and the shapes of words that surround them. In these examples, the illnesses are *not* substantially differentiated. They share two symptoms verbatim—"sleep problems" and "restlessness"—and each illness represents only a possible diagnosis based on a variety of affective experiences. Within textual representations of depression more generally, the two key elements of language and gender remain prominent, and the flexibility of definition—a flexibility that drug manufacturers capitalize on—appears integral to cultural understandings of the illness.

In the PaxilCR advertisement, even the words that are stacked upon each other, collectively referred to as "these symptoms of depression," avoid an absolute definition. The words atomize depression, drawing attention to elements of the illness experience that can make "life . . . feel difficult" and that therefore need remedying, but they do not exhaust the definitional possibilities. In fact, the word *depression* is used only once in the advertisement, as the object of the preposition in the phrase "symptoms of depression." The advertisement implies a definition of the illness (as the collection of the symptoms listed), but ultimately, it aligns its product with *any* combination of these symptoms—saying "if you have experienced *some of these symptoms* . . . you need relief" (emphasis added)—rather than with a single disease entity. This rhetorical move enables the drug to serve anxious and depressed populations equally, since what it offers is relief from a wide range of *symptoms* rather than a cure for a single *illness*. In fact, according to the FDA, Paxil is used to treat a range of mental illnesses: depression, panic disorder, social anxiety disorder, posttraumatic stress disorder, generalized anxiety disorder, and premenstrual dysphoric disorder. The interchangeability of the symptom words in the advertisements thus serves the marketing purpose of categorizing a range of *experiences* as problematic, and, in the process, it also promotes confusion about the boundaries of mental illnesses such as depression.

Even as readers are left wondering what combinations of symptoms might constitute a particular illness, the PaxilCR advertisement demonstrates the specifically linguistic nature of the experience of depression. The advertisement asks: "What's standing between you and your life?" It answers not, as expected, by naming depression itself, but graphically, by displaying the

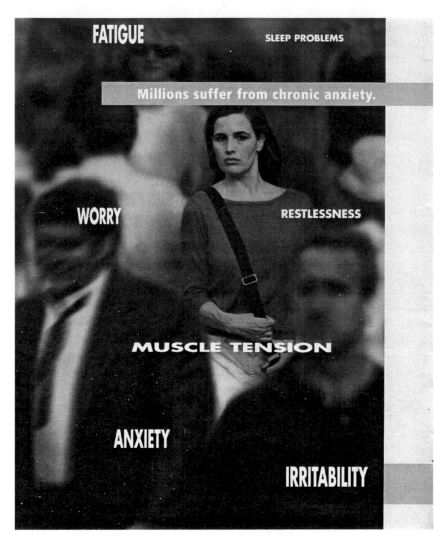

FIGURE 4. Paxil advertisement, 2001. (*New York Times Magazine*, October 28, 2001)

FIGURE 4. (continued)

FIGURE 5. PaxilCR advertisement, 2002. (*Time*, October 21, 2002, 67)

language of depression. Grammatically, nominalization renders each experience as a concrete symptom: "feeling depressed" becomes "depressed mood." Lexically, the choice of words to represent depression accommodates a broad and flexible definition. The list of symptoms excludes three—rapid weight changes, excessive guilt, and thoughts of death or suicide—that the American Psychiatric Association considers central to the illness.[20] Instead of providing the full list of symptoms, the advertisement highlights keywords that are applicable to a wide population, and it further translates medical terminology for symptoms (e.g., insomnia or hypersomnia) into more commonplace phrases (e.g., sleep problems). These translations, like the choice of which symptoms to include, address the broadest possible audience, but they also indict everyday experiences such as "restlessness" or "difficulty concentrating" as symptoms that demand treatment.

Experiences, rendered as symptoms, become the measures against which individuals are encouraged to measure their "health."[21] The tag line in both Paxil advertisements is: "Your life is waiting!®" Readers' lives, implicated by the second-person address, as well as those of the characters featured in the advertisements, exist beyond the bounds of their current expression of symptoms, and these lives can be retrieved in exchange for purchasing and ingesting the medication. As a registered trademark for Glaxo-SmithKline—a legal arrangement that gives the drug company ownership of this particular sequence of words—the sentence additionally stakes a claim to "your life." Having asserted its linguistic right to define a reader's "life" and its chemical power to deliver it, the Paxil advertisement directs attention toward the self, turning a voyeuristic impulse into an introspective one. It concludes with the command: "Talk to your doctor about . . . Paxil today. So you can see someone you haven't seen in a while . . . Yourself." As with the "life" waiting to be (re)claimed, the self is here made an object not currently possessed. It requires medical intervention to be seen. The advertisement encourages communication within the institutional space of a doctor's office, but this "talk" must be translated into a prescription before the self becomes visible again. Thus, the command to "talk to your doctor" occasions *more* language about mental health and illness, but it also directs the *content* of the conversation and implies the desired result.

Talk about "life" in the Paxil advertisements is transformed into talk about the drug, but this marketing strategy is predicated upon additional practices of self-monitoring (also encouraged by the advertisements) that lead individuals to their doctors' offices in the first place. The PaxilCR advertisement invites readers to observe others and then to reflect on their own "lives" and "selves." In this advertisement, the image is of others, but the bold text across the top of the page asks: "What's standing between *you* and *your* life?" (emphasis added). The interplay between the words, which expect an explanation from the reader, and the image, which portrays the isolation of the depressed woman, encourages introspection and comparison between the self and the image. As a result, the self is lost to the image. Below it, the text asserts: "Life is too precious to let another day go by feeling not quite 'yourself.'" At the end of the paragraph, in bold face, the advertisement promises: "Feeling balanced, more like 'yourself,' is within reach." The quotation marks—usually an indication of someone else's words, emphasis, or skepticism—around "yourself" suggest a curious self-consciousness in the use of the term. Either feeling like "yourself" is colloquial, and it is being quoted for authenticity, or it is a concept from which the text wishes to distance itself and its readers. In this second reading, "yourself" belongs in "scare" quotes because the "self," like the "life" promised in Glaxo-SmithKline's tag line, can be encountered only through Paxil. In other words, the quotation marks indicate a suspicion of the unmedicated self, and a promise of reclaiming the self (via medication) from an ambiguous illness identity. The twin abstractions—"life" and "self"—have become important commodities within direct-to-consumer pharmaceutical advertisements. Indeed, such texts do as much work policing the boundaries of what readers should expect of their lives (and of their selves) as they do identifying the medical conditions that the drugs purport to treat.

Within these definitions of "life" and "self," such texts focus attention on gender as a significant component of an illness identity. Both of these examples target women as potential patients, as do most advertisements for pharmaceuticals.[22] In the Paxil advertisement, the woman cannot blend into the crowd (she is not "going with the flow"); she is the object of the reader's scrutiny. She becomes—quite literally in the inset "after" photo at the bottom of the page—the "face" of chronic anxiety, and thus the advertisement offers an image of women as prone to the illness. In the PaxilCR advertisement, where "depression" (represented by its series of symptoms) stands between the woman and what appears to be her family, the clear implication is that a domestic life is what she should desire. Both she and her husband wear visible wedding bands, and in the small inset "after" photograph, the woman is reunited with her son, who leans on her shoulder. When depressed, the woman is a bad wife and mother; when cured, she returns to her familial place. The husband and father is curiously absent from the "after" photograph, which depicts only the woman and her son. His stance in the "before" photograph—both hands on his son's shoulders, weight on the leg farthest from his depressed wife—suggests his role as protector, but does little to suggest sympathy or caretaking. These empathetic roles appear to be reserved for the healthy wife and mother.

These images reinforce the textual claims of balance (emotional and chemical) achieved through pharmaceutical intervention and more clearly link illness to gendered identities. Reading the self through direct-to-consumer advertisements such as those for Paxil and PaxilCR reinforces conventional notions of gender: restlessness and agitation become depression in a wife and mother; worry and irritability become chronic anxiety in an unattached woman. In order for consumers to adopt one of these illness identities, they must, therefore, come to understand the self through the gendered lenses that the identities provide. These Paxil direct-to-consumer advertisements bring into focus a key insight about depression, namely, that words saturate images of the illness, but that they also divide, define, and isolate—fundamentally *shape*—the depressed individual, and, by extension, the "normal" self against which the depressed individual is defined. Language about depression originates in a variety of textual spaces including, but certainly not limited to, the marketing efforts of major pharmaceutical manufacturers. Indeed, the illness has become part of a public consciousness through a variety of outlets, including news reporting, government informational texts, memoirs, and other media. Together, such texts instantiate the discourse of depression; together, they offer a site for analyzing and understanding the linguistic means of articulating mental health and illness.

"Living under the Description" of Depression: The Language of Self-Doctoring

Antidepressant advertisements are arguments—they put forth an image of the healthy and the ill, reinforcing the contours of acceptable emotion and of threatening abnormality. The stakes of such discursive representations are high: people respond with acts of self-doctoring, literally serving as their own doctors and figuratively performing acts of self-fashioning that help them accommodate social expectations for such qualities as high energy, elevated mood, and uncomplaining caretaking. These practices are what Foucault calls "technologies of the self." They include "a certain number of operations on [individuals'] own bodies and souls, thoughts, conduct, and way of being, so as to transform themselves in order to attain a certain state of happiness, purity, wisdom, perfection, or immortality."[23] Such technologies of the self further rely on the forms of representation—verbal, physical, and textual—that individuals use in their gendered performances of health and illness. The linguistic habits of individuals—whether they compose lengthy memoirs or discuss their current litany of medications in the grocery line—clearly contribute to the popular understanding and experience of depression. In their repetition, statements identifying depression facilitate recognition of and regulate appropriate responses to the illness.

One might question, then, whether and how individuals shape these discursive practices. The notion that our statements might "speak us" rather than the reverse at first seems implausibly restrictive, yet we cannot deny that some statements—political stances, for example—entail far more than our simple declarative structures suggest. This sense of interconnectivity among statements is at the heart of theories of discourse. It also introduces the power of what Judith Butler calls "citationality," whereby the performative act is recognized less through individual intention than through successful *repetition or citation of a prior and authoritative set of practices*."[24] Accordingly, statements have power only insofar as they cite previous successful utterances. In this reading, the casual revelation of depression to a stranger while standing in the checkout line succeeds because it calls upon a number of other statements that have in the past achieved desirable social ends. The discourse of depression at the turn of the twenty-first century sanctions such statements because they are congruent with the notion of the illness as a troublesome biological malfunction rather than, as in previous eras, an intensely private psychological manifestation. Social connection may be achieved in the checkout line because it was already promised (in advertisements such as those discussed above) via pharmaceutical intervention. Such interactions are not, however, neutral. They compel the gendered self to monitor and regulate its activities in order to ensure its status as a legitimate source of successful statements of identity.

Viewing discourse as constitutive of gendered identities requires a theory of power and individual agency that is more flexible and nuanced than the common assumption of power as a unilateral imposition of force. For Foucault, in all "human relationships, whether they involve verbal communication . . . or amorous, institutional, or economic relationships, power is always present."[25] Yet this power should be understood as a series of ongoing, multidirectional, and mutable strategies, which can range from reasonably well-matched "strategic games" to outright "states of domination."[26] In between these two extremes are what Foucault calls "technologies of government," which mediate individuals' relationships with one another. Among these technologies are numerous "practices of the self," which feminist critics and others have suggested provide for a form of agency from within systems that makes change possible.[27] Significant change occurs only within the structures of discourse; it relies on the possibility that all statements and strategies are ultimately available for reappropriation. These strategies are particularly important in the late-modern period, when, according to Judy Segal, "lives [are] lived increasingly in the idiom of health and illness."[28] This "idiom" implies the contingent and discursive nature of health interactions, which depend on the language through which they are conducted. In response, a rhetorical approach to health-care practices—an individual and collective attention to the modes of persuasion available within medical encounters—reveals more dynamic relationships among actors, including both coercive and potentially empowering strategies. Such an approach, Segal suggests, "assumes and begins from complexity. A rhetorical analysis may not itself yield good medical advice, but it suggests a means of living with the fact that a revisable knowledge is medicine's only possible currency."[29] In other words, understanding health care in terms of "revisable knowledge" promotes a reflective and active engagement with the discourses that articulate states of health and illness. This engagement characterizes what I have been calling a rhetorical care of the self; it operates both within the "idiom of health and illness" and also from a critical distance that continually questions that idiom.

In the case of depression, the illness seems to resist such critical distance. According to the women I interviewed, talking with friends or counselors about feelings that might signal depression is difficult to do. Paige puts it simply: "when things are . . . such big problems that they need to be talked about, they're *too* big to be talked about." The women in both group interviews discussed strategies they used—describing their difficulties with "lack of motivation" or "stress"—to speak about their experiences, but the most common responses they report receiving are pamphlets about depression and drug information sheets. "The problem with those materials," Paige reports, is that "their solution is to . . . call that number and get drugs." Her skepticism of a pharmaceutical solution is, indeed, a place to locate a critical questioning of the discourse of depression, but she ends this conversational turn with a sigh and "so, I don't know," her voice trailing off. The women in Paige's group are equally limited in their own responses to the stories they hear from one another. After Claire tells the story of her mother's reaction—Claire reports her mother saying, "Why can't you just fix it yourself"—Su-Ting tentatively suggests "then maybe medication can help?" Claire agrees, immediately, that medication can help, "if you've got like a chemical imbalance." The simplicity of this pharmaceutical solution contrasts strongly with the women's other assertions about the difficulty of finding acceptable responses to and even willing conversational partners for their problems. Even in moments of critical distance, such as when Paige wishes for solutions *other* than drug therapies, the women have very few rhetorical tools with which to respond. All too soon, conversation returns to the language of biological psychiatry.

Emily Martin discovers a similar lack of rich vocabulary and rhetorical flexibility in her ethnography of manic depression support groups. The individuals she observes describe their mental states "within the narrow confines of categories—such as 'bipolar disorder' or 'depression'—whose terms are set by medical conventions such as the *DSM* and held in place by their required role in insurance claims, among other things. To my surprise," she writes, "I found that people in support groups used standard medical terms without further elaboration, frustrating my hope of finding rich, individually and culturally nuanced language about interior states."[30] This discursive conformity provides evidence of what Martin provocatively calls "living under the description of manic depression."[31] Rather than labeling individuals by their diagnosis, as is common among medical professionals, Martin's phrase "is meant to reflect the social fact that they have been given a diagnosis. At the same time, it calls attention to another social fact: the diagnosis is only one description of a person among many."[32] In addition, however, this phrase highlights the monological character of contemporary mental health discourse: lives are lived under psychiatric *descriptions*, rather than within the *dialogue* of pre-Prozac psychotherapy. This is not to suggest, necessarily, that such dialogue was somehow *better treatment*, but rather to point out that it constituted a more complex *rhetorical* situation through which mental health and illness emerged. Martin's frustration at the lack of individually meaningful representations of illness appears as an effect of the restricted discourse available and of a perceived need for universal categories of illness. The "shorthand" of clinical diagnoses assures common ground and allows for other kinds of performances of the self, but it also forecloses additional descriptions of health and illness. By accepting the diagnostic labels without qualification or modification—an act of linguistic self-doctoring—the support group members affiliate with the psychiatric institution and its current biological interventions.

In lieu of "individually and culturally nuanced language," Martin's project values other performances of "rationality" and "irrationality" from those living under the description of manic depression. Unquestionably, such alternative semiotic systems are at work, but to live under the description of an illness such as depression is to conform to prevailing ideas, to take up the circulating "idiom" in order to be recognized. This is certainly not a new phenomenon. Drawing on historical records, Andrew Solomon documents such adaptive behavior among seventeenth-century melancholics: "Two-thirds of the aristocrats who came to [a physician] complained of melancholy humors; and these men and women were well informed, speaking not simply of waves of sadness but complaining quite specifically on the basis of the scientific knowledge and fashion of the time. One such patient was 'desirous to have something to avoid the fumes arising from the spleen.'"[33] For these patients, the "scientific knowledge and fashion of the time" provided the language that made them recognizable to their physicians. Their reproduction of that language enabled them to receive treatment, but it also signaled their incorporation into a social discourse that associated melancholy with "great depth, soulfulness, complexity, and even genius."[34] Their performances were motivated by the desire to embody a poetic sensibility, rather than by the experience of illness. Such discursive manipulation represents active agency on the part of the patients (they secure a doctor's reception of their performance *as* melancholy, and they receive the treatments they seek), but it also represents their submission to a fashionable identity that had them ingesting concoctions that included "lapis lazuli, hellebore, cloves, [and] licorice powder . . . dissolved in white wine."[35] Their rhetorical performances entailed bodily interventions, not unlike contemporary doctors' visits that result in prescriptions for Prozac or Zoloft. The seventeenth-century patients' modeling of their talk on then circulating discourses constitutes a practice of self-doctoring aimed at achieving a particular social identity and resulting in significant physical treatments.

Such practices of self-doctoring provide evidence for a complex agency available to individuals. Rather than seeing individuals as mute and dominated subjects, feminist critics have attributed a "secret agency" to women as they take up the discourses surrounding femininity. Just as these discourses have been read to disempower women, medical discourses have traditionally been viewed as limiting patient agency. For women and patients, then, action must occur within an apparently dominating discourse. Women as "secret agents" perform beyond their surface femininity, which requires a disempowered subject. In addition to "the subject-in-discourse [who] is denied agency," there is "another subject who is here speaking in her capacity as a knowledgeable practitioner of the discourse of femininity."[36] In other words, a secret agency involves the skillful articulation of circulating discourses, rather than the attempt to liberate oneself from discourse per se; agency derives from the choices of citation made by individual subjects. This notion of a dual agency both submits individuals to circulating discourses (a patient's complaints must conform to familiar descriptions) and also performs within them to achieve individual ends, which mitigate the sense of disempowerment (the patient secures the intervention sought). Within the discourse of depression, such achievements often appear as practices of self-doctoring rather than as liberating or self-determined activities. Individuals perform their own diagnostic and curative activities, but in the process they alter their selves to accommodate the expectations and images encoded by the discourse. Self-doctoring, then, may achieve individual goals, but it does so at the expense of individual identities; it is often the practice of domination, rather than the participation in a strategic game.

Locating Possibilities for Self-Care

If self-doctoring too often deploys the "secret agent" in the service of submitting the self to biomedical interventions, the possibility of rhetorically richer engagements within the discourse of depression is nevertheless still available. Such a possibility resides in Foucault's notion of "curiosity," which, for him, "evokes the care one takes of what exists and what might exist; a sharpened sense of reality, but one that is never immobilized before it; a readiness to find what surrounds us strange and odd; a certain determination to throw off familiar ways of thought and to look at the same things in a different way; a passion for seizing what is happening now and what is disappearing; a lack of respect for the traditional hierarchies of what is important and fundamental."[37] Practices of self-doctoring ignore, among other things, the care of "what might exist"—a concern for possible futures—in favor of achieving immediate, instrumental ends. The possibility for "a lack of respect" for such established hierarchies, however, seems to be a compelling opening for a rhetorical care of the self that might challenge the dominant discourses and structures. Within the discourse of depression, "seizing what is happening now" might necessarily mean adopting some of self-doctoring's more coercive structures in order to be heard, but it might also mean resisting those structures ("a readiness to find" self-doctoring and pharmaceutical discourses "strange and odd," or "throwing off familiar ways of thought" in general), or at least deliberately deploying them toward one's personal ends. Drug-seeking behaviors among those who are not depressed could therefore be read as both a capitulation to the power of the pharmaceutical discourse and also as a rhetorical manipulation of the system (if they are successful). The ethics of such behavior are certainly complicated, but a self-conscious curiosity might enable individuals to act within the discourse of depression in more personally meaningful ways.

In volume three of his *History of Sexuality*, Foucault explores what he calls the "care of the self," which, he argues, arises in ancient Greek culture among a broader social practice of "self-cultivation." Such social practices encourage individuals to attend to their physical, moral, and spiritual health, as those concepts are defined by their culture. Such attention is not free, however, because it takes shape within the discourses of moral philosophy. Indeed, the "rapprochement . . . between medicine and ethics" provides "the inducement to acknowledge oneself as being ill or threatened by illness."[38] In other words, the self is constantly either actively ill or potentially so, resulting in self-fashioning activities that focus on healing or warding off illnesses. Such activities for Foucault are intrinsically social; they constitute "not an exercise in solitude, but a true social practice."[39] The social nature of practices of the self clarifies an important distinction between practices of self-doctoring (the submission of an isolated self to biomedical discourses and institutions) and a rhetorical care of the self (the critical examination of options and social positions for the self within discourse). My addition of the term *rhetorical* to Foucault's phrase is meant to signal this separation and to make room for practices of the self that acknowledge the situation of health and illness in language itself. Rhetorical criticism starts from an attention to situation and audience, and thus a *rhetorical* care of the self implies the conscious production of language and practice as a response to particular constellations of experience. Thus, a rhetorical care of the self is, indeed, an always already social endeavor, and it opens the possibility for conscious action and response to powerful discourses of health and illness.

To parse the complex relationships of power within the discourse of depression, I borrow a key distinction from Michel de Certeau between *strategies* and *tactics*. For de Certeau, the action of a secret agent might be labeled a *tactic*, a move which "must play on and within the terrain imposed on it and organized by the law of a foreign power."[40] A tactic does not operate from outside the dominant discourse, but it "takes advantage of 'opportunities' and depends on them. . . . It must vigilantly make use of the cracks that particular conjunctions open in the surveillance of the proprietary powers."[41] Such tactics are opposed to the *strategies* of powerful forces, in other words, the effects that institutions can impose upon others. De Certeau defines strategy as "the calculation (or manipulation) of power relationships that becomes possible as soon as a subject with will and power (a business, an army, a city, a scientific institution) can be isolated."[42] Specifically citing scientific institutions, de Certeau views strategies as the property of an entity that "postulates a *place* . . . with an *exteriority* composed of targets or threats."[43] A pharmaceutical company, for example, stakes its physical and intellectual territory—via patents, manufacturing sites, and trademarked language—from which it can deploy *strategies* such as advertisements and educational campaigns aimed at manipulating its target consumers. Within the discourse of depression, institutions aligned with biological psychiatry deploy strategies that encourage practices of self-doctoring, further subjecting individuals to pharmaceutical manipulations and self-definitions. Individuals, however, can counter such strategies via tactics that reclaim personal authority and challenge the dominant discourse. Such tactics participate in the rhetorical care of the self.

Practices of self-doctoring encompass activities that submit the self to further biomedical interventions and that shape it toward sanctioned gendered displays. Self-care requires countering tactics, which must grapple with the powerful primary texts that construct depression (for example, the *DSM*, direct-to-consumer advertisements, and even popular memoirs). In addition to individuals' tactics aimed at achieving personal goals and at challenging the dominant discourse, however, a rhetorical care of the self requires a counter-strategy located beyond the individual and grounded in an institutional context. Education and critique are strategies generated from institutions of school and, potentially, of medicine itself that offer the best chance for a care of the self rooted in strategic *curiosity*. Yet the contemporary discourse of depression is dominated by the institutions of biological psychiatry, which deploy strategies aimed at encouraging only practices of self-doctoring. One result of these strategies has been the narrowing of the linguistic field to a nearly monological engagement between the self and its brain chemistry. Patients become faulty machines; doctors become mechanics. To reverse this narrowing, a rhetorical care of the self advocates a self-conscious critique and skeptical orientation toward the dominant discourses of biological psychiatry. It advocates a dialogical relationship that attends to multiple texts and voices and that opens new possibilities for performances of the self and for definitions of mental health and illness. Such a rhetorical care of the self encourages and supports individuals' tactics, but it must also receive support from educational and medical institutions, which are in the position to deploy counter-strategies to make visible and accessible the opportunities for such tactics.

While activities participating in the rhetorical care of the self might, for a particular individual, result in a prescription for Prozac, that prescription emerges from a more complex and conscious series of rhetorical interactions than an identical prescription written in response to practices of self-doctoring. A rhetorical care of the self, then, does not liberate individuals from the discourse of depression; rather, it encourages them to engage in a dialogic relationship with that discourse and others. Rhetorical competency enables all of us to live consciously and carefully within the "idiom of health and illness." Such "tactical" moments within the late-modern discourse of depression reveal signs of self-care such as Paige's tentative skepticism about the solutions offered by drug information pamphlets. Nevertheless, much of the linguistic record—established through the print strategies of organized medical institutions and communities—demonstrates a restricted set of self-doctoring practices that maintain limited and gendered illness identities.

COMMANDING THEIR READERS to talk to their doctors, pharmaceutical advertisements attempt to restrict the content of those conversations to a narrow set of biological interventions. Beyond advertisements, pharmaceutical companies also produce materials targeting specific illnesses without mentioning their own drugs. For example, in October 1999 Pfizer placed a "patient education" insert in the *New York Times Magazine*, asserting that "Pfizer is helping millions of people realize that depression can be overcome." Offering additional "brochures about depression, its symptoms, and its treatment," the insert directs readers to http://www.depression-info.com. Such documents seem to promote self-care, since they do not overtly advertise a particular medication or prescribe a specific response to illness. Nevertheless, the corporate logo, copyright information, and the singular nominalization "treatment" strongly suggest the sort self-doctoring incentives a reader might find on the Web site.[44] Learning to read such texts—identifying the signs of corporate interests, for example—is an important step toward a truly rhetorical care of the self. This does not mean that individuals should discount all of the information Pfizer makes available, but it does suggest that a skeptical orientation—a curiosity— toward that information is necessary for a nuanced practice of self-care.

Such curiosity does exist, though my investigations suggest it is in need of nurturing, among consumers of such texts. Paige describes her conflicted responses to a Zoloft advertisement, saying "even when I identify with the Zoloft commercial . . . it also really pisses me off, because it's not like the guy who made that wants to get in my life and help me out. He wants to fucking sell me drugs, you know? Like, UAAGH!" She ends her statement with an inarticulate but highly expressive groan, vocalizing the difficulty of maintaining a curious stance toward the information presented by the pharmaceutical companies. Neither she nor the other women in the group remark on her assignation of a male gender to the institutional power behind the Zoloft advertisement.[45] Nevertheless, it is an important characterization: Paige clearly feels herself being patronized by the advice, and her response, although it fails to overcome the gendered power dynamic, suggests that she is not yet ready to comply with the advertisement's coercive message.

Elsewhere in our conversation, Paige performs a deconstruction of the link between pharmaceutical and "chemical depression," saying "a chemical process in the mind has something to do with the way I feel . . . but if you can convince yourself to be happy, there's a chemical process that goes with that . . . so it's a chemical solution the same as taking a pill." In these comments, Paige demonstrates a rhetorical awareness of the pharmaceutical companies' strategy of isolating "brain chemistry" as their sole province. She does not deny the possibility that such drugs might affect the way she feels, but she understands the mechanism of their action to be similar to the effects of something that resembles cognitive behavioral therapy as well. Her comments are dialogical, connecting to more than one framing discourse. While Paige and other readers must ultimately make choices that might even include accepting prescriptions for antidepressants, the presence of Paige's critical reading strategies suggests that a transformation of practices of self-doctoring into tactics for self-care is possible.

As various pharmaceutical campaigns demonstrate, self-doctoring includes a variety of tacitly *gendered* responses to depression and to one's social responsibilities in relation to mental health and illness. In the case of such texts, the discourse of depression can be seen not as incidentally *reflecting* but also as critically *shaping* the subjectivities that healthy and ill individuals have available to them. Linguistic structures, including the commands to "talk to your doctor," and rhetorical appeals, such as those to an idea of "social responsibility," fundamentally inform our concepts of health and illness, and they direct our actions in relation to those concepts. With the growth of the pharmaceutical industry and the popularity of biological psychiatry, concepts of health and illness have gradually constricted to focus on individuals' biochemistry. Many of the linguistic structures of the discourse of depression—including the definitions, metaphors, stories, and genres that textually represent the illness—display this narrowing and further direct self-doctoring practices toward biomedical activities and orientations toward the self. These structures not only represent but also constitute the experience of depression as "chemical imbalance," and they encourage the deployment of self-doctoring activities that respond to and validate this notion of the illness. Because such self-doctoring activities are embedded in language, the excavation work of close rhetorical analysis and critical reading promises to uncover the mechanisms by which they are naturalized. Further, such analytical strategies enact a rhetorical care of the self, which understands illnesses such as depression through *dialogical* rather than *monological* engagements with texts, scenes, and institutions. Mining the discourse of depression thus has the potential to reveal the linguistic promulgation of self-doctoring practices and also to uncover potential sites of rhetorical intervention, which may, in turn, translate into more fruitful health-care decisions for individuals. That is, rhetorical analysis helps us transform narrow practices of self-doctoring into a more diverse form of self-care.

3

Strategic Imprecision
and the Self-Doctoring Drive

In both medical and everyday practices, definitions of depression are often contingent and flexible, not necessarily adhering to the diagnostic precision that the *DSM* originally envisioned as its primary accounting goal. A certain amount of ambiguity and categorical expansion might be inevitable when interpreting the lived experiences of illness, but the discourse of depression maintains a *strategic* imprecision through a variety of linguistic and rhetorical structures. Such structures blur the boundaries between health and illness; they conflate experience and symptom, largely by deploying an apparently interchangeable vocabulary that has come to signify illness without specifying it. For individuals, this strategic imprecision results in self-doctoring practices that have the potential to overshadow necessary forms of self-care. Even the most cursory attention to the long historical record of depression and melancholia reveals a voluminous archive that similarly fails to circumscribe the illness. Robert Burton's *Anatomy of Melancholy*, published in five ever-expanding editions between 1621 and 1638, grows, as William Gass describes it, "from gigantic to gargantuan."[1] Burton's obsessive tinkering with and additions to his text reveal more than his personal fascination: his encyclopedic work collects folklore and mythology alongside the scientific discoveries of his era; it testifies to an already textually complex and rhetorically generative illness experience. Amid these multiple frames, depression exists as a more complex and multifaceted experience of the self than the contemporary discourse grants. In the late twentieth century, the popularity of memoirs, self-help guides, and academic studies of depression continues to reflect intense interest in the illness. But these texts heighten anxiety about the illness while nevertheless offering a very limited range of responses to it. In the collection of public texts that I assembled, consistently vague definitions of depression frustrate attempts to contain it. At first, this seems to counter the needs of biomedicine, where a precise definition would more accurately align with targeted pharmaceutical interventions. But, it quickly becomes clear that a strategic imprecision does more work than definitive definitions could in the service of encouraging pharmaceutical intervention. Self-doctoring practices emerge as natural responses to the discourse's fuzzy definitions, and these practices often result in prescriptions for medication rather than more accurate descriptions of the illness experience.

Situating depression as both normality and dysfunction, the discourse simultaneously supports two opposing understandings of the illness: that it is a severe medical condition ("clinical depression") and that it is a common emotional experience ("the blues"). As a result of this ambiguity, practices of self-doctoring attempt to locate the self via intense scrutiny of one's experiences and affects (and those of others), increased interactions with medical institutions, and heightened suspicion of all social interactions. Such practices of self-doctoring additionally work to gender depression by directing surveillance energies toward women's assumed greater emotionality and therefore their greater risk of illness.[2] With important consequences for both men and women, the multiple and changeable definitions of depression constitute not only the *occasion* but also the *compulsion* for self-doctoring. The linguistic and rhetorical foundations for this self-doctoring drive include depression's categorization as an *illness* rather than as a *disease*; its modification with a variety of qualifiers, such as *clinical* or *mild*; its differentiation from and affiliation with "the blues"; its inclusion in lists of common ailments; and its collocations with a gendered and at-risk self. These definitional practices invite *all* individuals to consider whether they, too, might be depressed.

What Is Depression?

Under the heading "What is a Depressive Disorder?" the NIMH general interest pamphlet, *Depression*, provides the following explanation: "A depressive disorder is an illness that involves the body, mood, and thoughts. It affects the way a person eats and sleeps, the way one feels about oneself, and the way one thinks about things. A depressive disorder is not the same as a passing blue mood. It is not a sign of personal weakness or a condition that can be willed or wished away. People with a depressive illness cannot merely 'pull themselves together' and get better. Without treatment, symptoms can last for weeks, months, or years. Appropriate treatment, however, can help most people who suffer from depression."[3] Of the seven sentences in this definition, the first two provide a vague description of the personal systems affected by the illness; the last two highlight the need for treatment; and the middle three focus on denying the idea that depression is related to normal sadness or a lack of willpower. None of these sentences, however, provides a definition of the illness itself. Instead, depression "involves" and "affects" individuals, who are encouraged to seek "appropriate treatment" to ease their suffering. In addition, because depression "involves the body, mood, and thoughts"—literally all physical and mental functions of an individual—it must be understood as affecting the very core of an individual's identity; indeed, it cannot be "willed or wished away"; it is part of the self. This paragraph aligns depression with the identities of the individuals who suffer from it, and it attempts to counteract particularly harmful responses to the illness (i.e., assuming depression is a "personal weakness"). Nevertheless, it fails to provide any specific symptoms beyond its broad generalizations, leaving readers without any more concrete knowledge than they had prior to reading it. That this is the first and only paragraph under the heading "What is a Depressive Disorder?" testifies to a general assumption that depression as illness needs little definitional attention. Readers' assumptions about *people* suffering from the illness are challenged by this paragraph, but their comprehension of *illness* remains unchallenged. Without elaboration of *how* depression is "not . . . a passing blue mood," readers have the freedom to draw their own conclusion about illness thresholds.

In a move that parallels the PaxilCR direct to consumer advertisement (figure 5) and other pharmaceutical marketing campaigns, the NIMH pamphlet text also implicates others beyond the depressed individual. In an earlier section of the pamphlet, the text asserts that "depressive illnesses cause pain and suffering not only to those who have a disorder, but also to those who care about them. Serious depression can destroy family life as well as the life of the ill person."[4] The audience for such a statement is curiously mixed. For those with depression, the statement reinforces social obligations and entailments—one is responsible not only for one's own illness, but for that illness's effects on others. For family and other readers with caretaking roles, this statement acknowledges suffering caused by extrinsic illness. Someone else's illness has the potential to "destroy family life." This being the case, *everyone* must be vigilant against an illness that remains opaque and poorly defined. The pamphlet's two persuasive moves—first that depression is an amorphous yet all-encompassing illness, and second that it harms not only individuals but entire social networks—encourage self- and other-monitoring as necessary forms of self-preservation. Such entailments, constructed within the discourse, also give the impression of an illness understood (how else could it be the object of surveillance?), while failing to demarcate its boundaries.

A broad and malleable definition of depression ensures that a wide range of individuals and experiences qualify for potential diagnosis. For mental health professionals, whose jobs require them to customize the definition of depression with each individual patient, policing the institutional boundaries of health and illness becomes a problematic endeavor. Their complex discursive negotiations reveal fault lines in the discourse of depression that are commonly submerged within the vague syntax of lay definitions. In my interview with mental health experts about their work with depressed patients, flexible definitions appear to be central to the therapeutic process. I asked the group to help me define depression, and their responses reflect the discourse's conflicting depictions of the illness. In the following excerpt, Joan, a social worker, responds first to my question "What is this thing we call 'depression'?":

JOAN: Well, I think it is easy to talk about depression in a way that doesn't necessarily have like a *clinical* component, but sort of is still valid. I mean, I know in terms of the kids that I've worked with, and the settings that I've worked on, we definitely had kids who were diagnosed as depressed. But, then, we also saw lots of kids who weren't really that happy, but they weren't depressed. And so, I don't know. It's easy, . . . aside from professional life, to understand what that [i.e., depression] means, or to have, I guess, a sense of what that means, without necessarily meaning what it means in the *DSM-IV*. That's my initial reaction to that question.

For Joan, and for many others, depression can be divided into two phenomena: a clinical entity and a more amorphous social experience that is both quite common and less diagnosable within institutional guidelines. Joan struggles to see both forms of depression as "valid," acknowledging that a clinical diagnosis applies only to a subset of the children with whom she has worked. Other children's unhappiness, however, qualifies as a form of depression associated with life "aside from professional life." Moments later, Joan returns to this binary construction suggesting that clinical depression might indeed be chemically based and, therefore, might respond to antidepressants. But other kinds of depression, she asserts, are more likely related to stressful life events and to require social interventions. This second form of depression seems to be an expanding category that bears an uncertain relationship to "professional diagnoses" of illness that label some individuals. The depression that is not clinically validated nevertheless causes suffering and deserves treatment, but Joan comprehends it primarily intuitively rather than systematically. In Joan's binary system, the stability and validity of a clinical diagnosis is assumed, but for the other mental health professionals, all of whom have had much more clinical experience with depressed individuals, a tactical imprecision—one that allows therapeutic flexibility—resides within practices of professional diagnosis as well. Ellen, a psychiatrist, speaks next:

ELLEN: I agree that you see a lot of different faces of depression. And I always have to clarify with people. It's one of the things I do the first time I see them, is to find out what they mean when they tell me they're depressed. And, frequently they have a hard time describing that. But for a lot of people, being depressed means they're just not interested in things, and they're generally slowed down and feeling dead. And then there's a huge percentage of people who are actually feeling guilty and can't stop thinking about all of the things that they think that they have done and how they're a really horrible person, and so there's a lot of self-blame that goes into it. And some people feel sad. And all of that goes in to their subjective feeling of depression. But I'm also looking for objective things, like their sleep, their appetite, their social interactions, their ability to experience pleasure, and how persistent that is throughout their day. Does their mood respond? Or does it not respond? Is their mood variable depending upon the time of day? Or, you know, if they win the lottery, are they going to feel happy? Or are they still going to just [say] "I can't imagine what I would do; I'd still have to kill myself." So, I think it's very variable what people mean when they say they're depressed.

Ellen describes a variety of affective states that count as depression for the people with whom she interacts. She generalizes from her clinical experience and offers a composite picture of the depressed individual as "generally slowed down and feeling dead," as "feeling guilty," and as exhibiting persistent changes in behavior and affective experience. Yet, even though such a template is readily accessible for Ellen, she says she must find out from each patient "what they mean when they tell me they're depressed." Elsewhere in the interview, she describes her patients' surprise at her need to establish a definition of depression with their input. They assume that the concept is stable and universal; they enter her office having already performed their own self-diagnosis; they are seeking treatment. Ellen says, "[When] I was first starting out, and I would say [to patients] well, you know, what does that [i.e., depression] mean to you? It seemed like a lot of people would get sort of put off by that and say, 'Well, I'm depressed. Don't you know what that means?'" Ellen's encounters with patients taught her to ask the question in more circuitous ways, including asking patients how they know that they are *becoming* depressed. Directing her patients' attention away from a present assertion of illness and toward a progressive self-evaluation, Ellen's question views depression as an evolving experience rather than as a singular identity ("I am depressed"). She is, in effect, inviting her patients to engage in a rhetorical care of the self—to attend to a personal definition of health and/or illness—rather than to receive the treatment dictated by their practices of self-doctoring. The conflict that arises for patients who are asked to define their illnesses in this way reveals a widespread belief that the illness is consistent and stable. Yet, in Ellen's words, "It's very variable what people mean when they say they're depressed." For Ellen, individual definitions take precedence over clinical or professional diagnoses, but her practice runs counter to the stereotypical assurance of medical expertise assumed by Joan's assertion of a clinical depression "meaning what it means in the *DSM-IV*."

For readers of texts such as the NIMH brochures, depression appears on the surface to be a stable, unified illness, but the definition encompasses a wide range of potential experiences, which can be read into the definition from individuals' lives. This reading of the self into an available illness identity is the most powerful of the discursive self-doctoring practices. After recognizing themselves in the definition of the illness, individuals are understandably surprised by doctors who do not immediately perform the same interpretive act. They might even—as Ellen implies—be put off by doctors who ask them to examine their own self-diagnosis. Ellen's description of her practice, especially her frank admission that her patients at first doubted her credibility when she did not immediately validate their self-diagnoses, draws attention to the power of the discourse of depression, which convinces individuals they have an illness even when they cannot precisely define it.

For Laurie, a clinical psychologist, and Betty, a psychiatric nurse, this definitional imprecision leads to conflicts between patients' realities (they understand themselves to be depressed) and their potential diagnoses.

BETTY: Yeah, I have a lot of people that come in and tell me that they are depressed, but when I run through the *DSM-IV* diagnoses or symptoms with them, they don't even qualify as dysthymic [a less serious but chronic form of depression], sometimes. But they feel depressed, and that doesn't qualify as a diagnosis or as eligible for medications However, I have friends who I would consider not depressed who are on the medications=

JOAN: =absolutely=

ELLEN: =oh yeah=

BETTY: =so, [laughs] I don't know, I guess it depends on who you are and what insurance you have and=

LAURIE: =what system you're in=

BETTY: = [overlapping] what system you're in

JOAN: = [overlapping] absolutely

LAURIE: Mmmm hmmm. Yeah, I mean I see that. I mean, I have a lot of friends who I don't consider depressed at all. Not a lot, I have some. And I also have seen some of my clients that probably aren't depressed, but they have a really good insurance, and until that runs out, they will be able to get therapy for what they want. Well, I should take, I (need to) go backwards. They are depressed. But they're not of sufficient depression to qualify under *DSM*. But they're depressed. They're unhappy with their lives. I mean there is something in their life that's making them sad and all, but do they probably need to be on the meds? And . . . for me is there good clinical evidence that they ought to be on meds? No.

Both Betty and Laurie relate stories of individuals who do not seem to meet the standards for a clinical diagnosis, but who are nevertheless receiving medication and/or therapy for depression. Both Joan and Ellen indicate agreement in several affirmative latching phrases (e.g., Ellen's "oh yeah" that follows without pause after Joan's first "absolutely") and overlapping minimal responses (e.g., Joan's second "absolutely" that overlaps Betty's turn). It is hardly news that there might be disparities in access to health care, but these anecdotes point to an important facet of the discourse of depression. The rhetorical force of an individual's self-diagnosis depends on her or his social and economic status and access to particular forms of care: Laurie's patients are part of her private clinical practice; Betty's seek care through local hospitals. Beyond this unfortunately predictable disparity, however, lies another important discursive reality, namely, that self-diagnosis occurs prior to clinical diagnosis. In addition, depression has become a touchstone for seeking medical—primarily pharmaceutical—intervention. Laurie sees little "clinical evidence that [her patients] ought to be on meds," but many of them are nonetheless. They are "on meds" because they have accepted illness identities that fault their brain chemistry for their unhappiness.

Patients may respond to imprecise definitions of illness by reading themselves into the illness identity provided, but these mental health professionals use imprecision in more tactical ways; they turn the discursive strategy into therapeutic interventions. In Ellen's clinical practice, the definition of depression must be negotiated and articulated individually by each patient; for Laurie and Betty, having good insurance may mean receiving treatment for what might technically be categorized as "subclinical" depression, but which nevertheless deserves intervention, though both seem skeptical as to the value of *pharmaceutical* intervention. Within my corpus, a variety of definitional practices maintain a porous border between "clinical" and "normal" depressions, encouraging reading practices that classify a wide range of experiences as problematic, indeed, symptomatic. While the mental health professionals may seek to transform such self-doctoring into forms of self-care, their efforts must acknowledge and resist the powerful discourse that shapes the identities of patients who seek their help and intervention. Examining definitional practices within the discourse of depression, therefore, becomes a first step toward understanding and, perhaps, making tactical use of these illness identities. Patients who enter the medical encounter understanding themselves to be depressed—both Ellen's who must articulate the boundaries of their particular depressions, and Betty's who fail to meet the *DSM* diagnostic criteria—are surprised to encounter a new negotiation of meaning with these mental health professionals. To have placed themselves in this situation, such patients have already adopted the illness identity dictated by the discourse. Whether or not they qualify for treatment and insurance reimbursement, they have come to understand and define themselves as depressed. They do so in response to the language through which the illness is communicated, language that transforms experiences into symptoms and people into patients.

"Semantic Damage": The Vocabulary of Illness

Railing against terminology forms one consistent response to depression, a response that indicates frustration with available illness identities and also the social responses to them. William Styron famously accused *depression* of having "usurped" the lexical place once occupied by *melancholia*, "a far more apt and evocative word."[5] He condemns *depression*, which "has slithered innocuously through the language like a slug, leaving little trace of its intrinsic malevolence and preventing, by its very insipidity, a general awareness of the horrible intensity of the disease when out of control."[6] The violent revulsion with which Styron describes the word reflects his sense of disconnection and alienation from others; he blames his experience partially on the language rather than his illness. Accusing the scientist who first used *depression* to name the clinical phenomenon of inflicting "semantic damage," Styron suggests that such rhetorical choices amount, essentially, to euphemistic camouflage that hinder acknowledgment and, perhaps, treatment of the illness.

Despite the poetic resonance of its disdain, Styron's accusation only partially accounts for the historical record of the term, which has encompassed multiple meanings for centuries. The word came into the English language in the fourteenth century as an astronomical term meaning "the angular distance of a star . . . below the horizon." By 1533, it had acquired the meaning of "being brought low," and by 1665, the term was in use to refer to a "great depression of spirits." In the early twentieth century, the term is indeed, as Styron points out, applied professionally to a clinical phenomenon; this technical definition exists alongside a variety of other meanings. From economic ("a downturn in finances") to geographic ("a low place"), such meanings remain available in the current lexicon and dilute the severity of the medical application. Nevertheless, the semantic problem that Styron identifies arises not from the word itself, nor even from its use in diagnostic settings, but rather from a collection of everyday discursive practices that actively resist a singular, precise definition of depression.

Perhaps counterintuitively, such practices include the very definitional strategies that attempt to codify the experience of illness. For example, modification—pairing *depression* with intensifiers such as *severe*, *chronic*, or *clinical*—appears to offer subcategories of depression (and therefore precision), but a close examination fails to establish clear systemization among the adjectives. Similarly, contrastive statements emphasize that depression *is not* the common experience of sadness, yet in making such claims, they ensure that depression and sadness inhabit the same lexical field. Finally, analogous reasoning places depression alongside other recognized and serious diseases, asserting parity between the named entities; but this practice ignores the dissimilarities in function and form that complicate such comparisons. In each of these strategies, depression becomes visible not as a single entity or illness, but rather as the *problem* of delimiting a set of experiences as abnormal or unexpected. Indeed, the illness becomes visible only when an individual's "normal functioning" has been disrupted. Thus, depression exists always in relationship to everyday activities and experiences. Titling his memoir *Malignant Sadness*, Lewis Wolpert implies that "normal sadness is to depression what normal growth is to cancer."[7] Yet, whereas cancer has been divorced from its relationship to normal cell growth, the phrase "malignant sadness" literally encompasses the nonmedical experience of sadness, even as it attempts to define depression *against* that experience. Ultimately, such coinages serve to reinforce the status of depression on a continuum with healthy emotions, and, as a consequence, to maintain the semantic imprecision against which Styron rails. Rather than lament this state of affairs, however, we might try to understand this flexibility—and the definitional strategies that enact it—as an important determinant of the available illness identities. Seen in this way, the lack of a precise definition for depression becomes a significant actor, encouraging practices of self-doctoring among both healthy and ill individuals.

First-person narrative texts about depression offer a response to the bodily disruption of illness.[8] Yet, unlike many illness narratives such as those about cancer that most often center on the moment of discovery or diagnosis—an event that organizes life into before and after, into *health* and *illness*—depression narratives iteratively return to such definitional moments, always resisting and questioning them. Defining depression and thereby containing it is rarely a straightforward or singular process in recent memoirs of the illness. In *Willow Weep for Me* (1999), Meri Nana-Ama Danquah admits her depression to a friend, Jade, who also suffers from depression. Danquah describes her discomfort with the label "clinical depression," which she has recently heard attached to herself. Jade responds: "As far as I'm concerned . . . all depression is clinical. People who are just having a bad day should use another word. They shouldn't say stuff like 'I'm so depressed because I failed a test' or 'I broke my nail and I'm depressed.' They're not depressed. They don't even begin to understand what real depression is."[9] Echoing Styron, Danquah's friend wishes the term *depression* could be restricted in everyday use. Quoting unnamed others who use the term for what she considers to be trivial incidents, Jade exemplifies another rhetorical facet of the definition of depression, namely, that it forms in opposition to utterances deemed inadequate. Her call to "use another word" for these incidental frustrations and painful experiences—much like Styron's nostalgic yearning for a return to the use of *melancholia*—might be seen less as a commentary on semantic paucity than as central to the definition of depression itself. Her formula—X is not real depression—recurs throughout the discourse, nevertheless maintaining the link between X (a common experience) and depression itself. Danquah herself questions the notion of a "real depression" even as her friend asserts it. "What is real depression?" she asks, "How did you know that's what you were feeling?"[10] Danquah's uncertainty about the definition of depression turns quickly into doubt first of her friend ("How did you know") and then of herself. Her identity reflects the strategic imprecision of depression's definition—left uncertain about the boundaries of illness, she turns her gaze inward, toward introspection and self-monitoring.

For Elizabeth Wurtzel, the search for a definition takes place through a series of ultimately inadequate comparisons. In *Prozac Nation* (1994), she tries to find a semantic approximation for her experience, but eventually settles for just "this," a pronoun without a clear antecedent. She writes of her adolescent experiences with depression:

> Here was this thing called depression that was not definable in any sort of concrete way (was it bigger than a breadbox? smaller than an armoire? animal, vegetable, or mineral?) that had simply taken up residence in my mind—a mirage, a vision, a hallucination—and yet it was creeping into the lives of everyone who was close to me, ruining them all as I was ruined myself. If it were a pestilence, like the roaches that used to creep around the kitchen of our apartment, we could have called an exterminator; if it were a fire, we could have turned an extinguisher on it; my God, even if it were something simple like having trouble with quadratic equations in algebra class, there were tutors who could have taught me about $2ab$ or 3^2 or how to mix numbers and letters so they are just right. But this was just madness. I mean, I wasn't an alcoholic, an anorexic, a bulimic, or a drug addict. We couldn't blame this all on booze or food or vomit or thinness or needles and the damage done. My parents could argue until late into the night about what to do about *this*—this thing— but they were basically bickering about something that in measurable terms did not exist.[11]

"This thing"—Wurtzel's depression—resists her attempts at quantification; it cannot be articulated in concrete terms. Wurtzel resorts to a series of ephemeral descriptors—mirage, vision, hallucination—and then to a series of violent analogies, signaling her increasing frustration at finding no clear imagery. Wishing, by extension, to exterminate, to extinguish, or even simply to educate her way out of depression, Wurtzel relies on the domestic scenes of her childhood to situate her illness. Failing to identify it within the household and scholastic worlds of her youth, she moves to a series of diagnostic labels for her *self*, eventually rejecting alcoholism, anorexia, bulimia, and addiction, as well as their attendant practices and crutches, as possible models for her experience. Left with the conclusion that her illness "in measurable terms did not exist," Wurtzel cries out for "a real ailment."[12] A real illness, she concludes, would not exist merely as a series of negative propositions, but would take shape within visible, measurable boundaries and in the production of recognizable actions. Failing on both counts, depression constitutes a problematic relationship between Wurtzel and her self. The relationship ultimately transfers the problem of definition from the illness to the self, particularly the female self, since scenes of self-questioning such as Danquah's and Wurtzel's are more common to women's memoirs.

Wurtzel's series of negative propositions also makes use of analogical reasoning to attempt to define her experience. Wurtzel's rejected ailments begin to situate depression alongside other, presumably more accessible illnesses and identities. For Martha Manning, such comparisons are all too easy to perform. In her memoir, *Undercurrents* (1995), she describes the advice-giving impulses of well-meaning but inadequately informed friends and acquaintances. She writes: "People hear the word *depression* and figure that since they've felt down or blue at some point in their lives, they are experts, which is like assuming that because you've had a chest cold, you are now qualified to treat lung cancer."[13] For Manning, a faulty analogy serves as enough authority for nondepressed individuals to speak as "experts," even to "treat" illness. Here, the self-doctoring drive transforms into other-doctoring as friends and acquaintances attempt to provide her with their own brands of medical advice. Manning's argument against such practices rests on the negative proposition— she rejects the common assumption that depression is related to everyday sadness and in the process aligns depression with cancer, just as Wolpert does in his choice of a title.

Although appeals for equality between physical and mental illnesses are important factors in gaining access to and reimbursement for health care, they nevertheless rest on simple correlations between measurable physical attributes—glucose levels or blood pressure readings—and mental experiences that are, unfortunately, unquantifiable, and accessible only through the language used to describe them. Even as comparisons between, for example, depression and cancer attempt to clarify depression's status as disease, they introduce new expectations for precise measurement and evaluation. These expectations run counter to the pressures of the discourse of depression, which consistently denies precision and heightens anxieties about illness boundaries. Thus, the discourse encourages self-doctoring first by obscuring depression's threshold and then by offering only partially successful analogies with physically measurable illnesses. In first-person memoirs, expressions of frustration, anxiety, and anger testify to these discursive pressures. Ultimately, though, they present few alternatives to the definitional practices provided in other public texts. In the public informational texts I collected, linguistic strategies of definition—including classification, modification, differentiation, and analogy—confuse rather than clarify depression's boundaries. Further, these discursive practices produce the need for self-doctoring as a response to a nearly universal risk of illness.

Depression Is Not a Disease

At the core of definition lies a need to classify, to collect like-featured items into groups. For depression, a classification more basic than any included in the *DSM* is the distinction between *illness* and *disease*. In my corpus, depression most often falls into the former category, but other labels such as *condition*, *disorder*, and *disease* are sometimes attached to it.[14] Each of these terms classifies depression in a different way, framing it within cultural, social, and biological models of experience. The primary distinction—between the terms *illness* and *disease*—produces significant cultural critiques and shapes the possible rhetorical effects of labeling oneself *depressed*. According to Arthur Kleinman, the term *illness* "refers to how the sick person and the members of the family or wider social network perceive, live with, and respond to symptoms and disability."[15] This definition carries deeply social, cultural implications that justify extensive interpretive attention. *Disease*, on the other hand, is "an alteration in biological structure or functioning," a definition that excludes the meanings made out of experience.[16] Following from Kleinman's distinction, *illness* requires social judgment and response, whereas *disease* remains a structural and ostensibly objective phenomenon. The transition from disease to illness occurs only, as Christopher Boorse argues, "through normative judgments" and through the "activat[ion] of social institutions."[17] In other words, *disease* must be accompanied by social judgment before it constitutes *illness*.

Furthermore, *ill* as an adjective describing health refers to being "unsound, disordered," but *illness* historically evoked a secondary meaning of "wickedness, depravity; evil conduct; badness." Since the eighteenth century, English has substituted *badness* to refer to the most of the pejorative senses of *illness*, but the term's early associations are retained in such words as *ill-tempered*, *ill-advised*, *ill-bred*, and *ill-conditioned*, each of which implies moral judgment and individual culpability. By contrast, *disease* refers to "a departure from the state of health, especially when caused by structural change," a definition that exonerates individuals from responsibility for their experience.[18] While sickness in general—whether disease or illness—is negative departure from "normal" health, the responses to and tolerance for it depend in part on how it is classified. Diseases incur prescribed responses and follow known courses; illnesses are more uncertain and occasion heightened social negotiation and monitoring. A disease model of depression appears to suit pharmaceutical companies—their medications are ideal packaged responses—so the insistence in the discourse on naming depression an *illness* represents an important divergence from a narrowly biochemical disease model. Nevertheless, pharmaceutical rhetoric supports this imprecision precisely because it implicates *more* individuals as potentially ill. Drawing attention to problematic social interactions (as opposed to malfunctioning bodies), the term *illness* encompasses a wider range of behaviors and experiences, therefore expanding the potential patient population.

Two related terms, carrying social implications similar to those of *illness* are also common as referents for depression: *condition* "a particular mode of being of a person or thing," and *disorder* "a disturbance of the bodily (or mental) functions." *Condition* parallels *illness* in its social and euphemistic connotations: to be "in a certain, delicate, interesting, or particular condition" can refer to pregnancy or to another health status about which circumspection is assumed to be required. *Disorder* substitutes for *disease*, without implying the structural causality for the breakdown. It frequently refers to mental functions, thus distancing it from the biological, systemic interpretation common to the term *disease*. Returning to depression, we must conclude, with Lewis Wolpert, that "it is hard to think of mental illnesses in the same way as [we] think about heart disease or cancer. . . . Illness is a combination of symptoms and signs."[19] *Illnesses* can be multiply read via their symptoms and signs; they are social entities. When it is seen as an *illness*, depression is subject to a potentially contradictory set of readings and judgments. While the tenets of biological psychiatry seem to dictate the disease model of brain chemistry, the discursive preference for *illness* ensures that depression remains a primarily social phenomenon, one that requires a range of regulatory responses.

The discourse encourages regulation, particularly self-regulation, in responses to illness, and it therefore shapes possible illness identities through these behaviors. Attempts to disentangle illness from identity, in effect to make depression a *disease*, fail within the contemporary discourse. For Peter Kramer, messy, cultural beliefs about depression—including, presumably, the fluid vocabulary through which it is described—hinder the aggressive treatment of the disease. It is strange, then, that he both acknowledges and ultimately ignores the power of terminology in constituting this reality for the illness. He writes in his preface to *Against Depression*: "About word choice: For the most part, I honor the distinction between *disease*, a pathological condition of an organism, and *illness*, the poor health that results from disease. But I am not overly scrupulous about this distinction, a tendency that I think is excusable in the case of what we call a mental illness, where we mean a disease that affects the mind."[20] Kramer "honors" the distinction between pathology (disease) and poor health, defined as the social effects of pathology (illness); but he suggests that this is more for the sake of convention than any conviction that the two labels and the phenomena that they describe might result in disparate analyses. His justification—that "what we call mental illness" is both a disease and its results, illness—rests on the assumption that the "mind" is social and diseases that affect the mind are therefore also illnesses. Yet Kramer's text makes the argument that we ought to oppose depression vigorously and unequivocally, based on the assertion that it is a *disease* in the biological/functional respect. The laxity about terminology that he admits to and seems unconfined by nevertheless reinforces the cultural paradigm that he has set himself against. If depression is at least in part a social condition, then it cannot be eradicated with a science-fiction wonder drug (as Kramer suggests in his book's central thought experiment); if it is socially constructed and experienced, it cannot be treated simply by standing "against" it. Indeed, Kramer's book, despite attempting to argue for a new conception of depression, fails to achieve either the semantic shift or the attending conceptual shift from *illness* to *disease*. Kramer is by no means alone in his lexical conflations: as an analysis of contemporary texts about depression demonstrates, definitions of depression are systematically imprecise.

In my corpus, depression is overwhelmingly classified with the term *illness* (see table 3.1). To illustrate this finding, the phrase *mental illness* occurs eighty-five times, while the phrase *mental disease* occurs only once in the nearly 240,000 words. This suggests what we ultimately know: depression is discussed in social rather than purely biological terms. Considering it an *illness* focuses attention on the affective status of sufferers and the meanings made of their experiences. The model for *disease* is one of a course of treatment and cure; a structural anomaly is fixed and the patient returns to a "healthy" state.

TABLE 3.1

Frequency of Classificatory Terms for Depression in the Corpus

	Total Occurrences	*Defining Depression*	*Percentage of Total Definitions*
Illness	266	210	52.50
Disorder	386	118	29.50
Condition	93	51	12.75
Disease	148	21	5.25
Total	893	400	

SOURCE: Examples taken from research corpus of contemporary language about depression (1995–2005).

An *illness*, however, generates multiple meanings. In her memoir, *The Beast: A Journey through Depression* (1996), Tracy Thompson struggles with the word *illness*, calling it a "concept that had layers of meaning. There was illness that was caused by something you could see, if only under a microscope, like the bacterium that caused tuberculosis—or it was something whose effects were visible, like cancer. Then there was another kind of illness, as in, 'God, she's a sick person,' 'How sick,' 'This is a really sick idea.' The second kind carried the weight of moral blame. There was an element of choice involved—or, if not choice, some residual notion of original sin."[21] For Thompson, *illness* reintroduces the element of personal responsibility for her own depression; it carries the taint of "sin" and the implication of having somehow chosen to be ill.

Further, *illness* implies a whole identity—as in "she's a sick person"—for Thompson. Similarly, the term *condition* implies an identification between self and disease. In the NIMH pamphlet *Depression: A Treatable Illness*, the text asserts that depression "is not a sign of personal weakness or a condition that can be willed or wished away."[22] Here, the term *condition* accompanies both *weakness* and a failure of *will*. And, while this is a definition by denial rather than by affirmation, depression itself is still the antecedent for both *condition* and *sign*, which situates it in social and interpretive, rather than objective, realities. As written in one *Newsweek* article, Elizabeth Wurtzel's "success" does not "mitigate her basic condition. Her face is drawn and long strands of hair have come loose from her untidy blond bun."[23] Here, Wurtzel's depression defines her whole being; it is her basic condition. It is also a condition defined exclusively by her physical appearance, drawing parallels between her "untidy" hair and an implied disorganized identity. This definitional moment not only aligns Wurtzel herself with depression, it also works toward gendering the illness by attending to feminized features such as her "blond bun."

Echoing Wurtzel's untidiness, the classification of *disorder* is more common than its more straightforwardly biological cousin *disease*. For example, in a *Blues Buster* article, depression is defined as "a disorder of mind and body."[24] The term *disorder* gives a general sense of disorganization and disruption. Its use is qualitatively different from instances of *disease*, which often collocate with concrete social actions and responses. When *disease* does define depression, it is generally paired with concrete, finite actions, for example: "Margaret Ann Aitcheson was hospitalized more than once with the disease."[25] Here, the action of hospitalization seems to trigger the use of the term *disease*. In other cases, *disease* appears because it is in the same lexical field as another term in the sentence, as in "[d]epression is not . . . a disease that you caught somehow."[26] In this case, depression assumes the label of *disease* only tangentially: it is distanced from the label both by the negative construction and by the analogy, which requires *disease* because biological agents spread contagions that may be "caught." Significantly, of the twenty-one instances of *disease* specifically defining depression, five (24 percent) occur in articles commenting on childhood depression. Perhaps because children are assumed to be less responsible for their maladies, their experiences of depression are easier to characterize as the result of biological malfunction. Within my corpus, depression emerges as a complex social illness, one that requires significant self-monitoring to recognize and ameliorate. The consistent use of *illness* as a classificatory term reinforces these self-doctoring pressures and establishes the need for further definitional moves.

Modifiers That Multiply Depressions

Beyond its broad classification as an illness, depression receives a variety of additional qualifiers that seem at first to offer more precision. Among them, the most common are *major* depression, *serious* or *severe* depression, and *clinical* depression (see table 3.2). Yet each of these terms, even as it attempts to catalog versions of the illness, multiplies the possibilities without clarifying the underlying entity. *Major* depressions usher in the possibilities of *minor* ones; *serious* depressions imply nonserious, even potentially mundane counterparts; *clinical* depressions indicate a range of illnesses that are properly handled outside the medical system. In each case, an intensifier realizes not a single form of illness, but multiple forms. As a consequence of this proliferation, overlapping near-synonyms (*serious, severe; mild, minor; disabling, debilitating*) do little to help divide the illness into meaningful categories. Indeed, the presence of *normal* as a modifier of depression signals not just category expansion but also the possibility that at least *some* depressions are not illnesses at all. The availability within the discourse of so many species of depression produces myriad illness

TABLE 3.2

Modifiers for Depression in the Corpus

Modifier	No.	Modifier	No.	Modifier	No.
Major	136	Psychotic	6	Moderate	36
Severe	58	Disabling	3	Mild	21
Clinical	29	Incapacitating	3	Minor	6
Serious	21	Debilitating	2	Normal	6

SOURCE: Examples taken from research corpus of contemporary language about depression (1995–2005).

identities—perhaps one for every depressed individual—but they are identities that must constantly justify their status as illnesses lest they be judged *minor*, *mild*, or, simply, *normal*.

In use, these modified forms of depression create anxiety for individuals, who often wish to avoid an illness identity altogether. Danquah describes her distress at being labeled by a friend as "severely depressed." She writes: "If he had just said he thought I sounded depressed, I think I would have been able to handle that because the word, depression, is thrown about casually to describe moods that are relatively normal in the scale of human emotions. What I found distressing was that he qualified it as *severe*."[27] Similarly, Manning responds several times to the intensifiers applied to her condition: "She tells me that I am 'quite depressed.' I can tolerate being labeled 'depressed.' 'Quite depressed' sounds more serious and feels 'quite' uncomfortable when applied to me"[28] and "I keep trying to label my experiences with depression as *episodes*, but they keep using words like *chronic, recurrent, and cyclic*. I hate their words. I want my depression to be over, totally and completely over."[29] For both women—and these statements occur most often in women's memoirs—the modification of depression signals an inescapable illness identity rather than an emotional state. Danquah and Manning both accept, even expect, a level of depression in their lives; to begin to view themselves as ill, however, they must hear themselves labeled with *more* than just depression. This seems to be a distinction common to women's memoirs but not to men's, in which the *fact* of depression is more salient than the *degree*. Women's identities are already at risk for depression; to qualify as ill, a woman's depression must be qualified by an intensifier. For men, the discourse offers a different form of gender identity: to be depressed at all risks feminization and is therefore already distressing enough to count as illness.

Part of depression's close association with women undoubtedly arises from the unique forms of the illness linked to women's reproductive cycles. Discussions of menstruation and childbirth sometimes blur the boundaries between normal emotional responses and illness identities for women at these life stages. In a *Newsweek* article about postpartum depression (PPD), a "normal" mother with PPD is compared to Andrea Yates, who in 2001 drowned her five children while she was apparently suffering postpartum psychosis (PPP). The comparison is clearly meant to differentiate *depression* from *psychosis*, yet the syntax suggest another reading, one that suspects all mothers of potential violence and uncontrollable emotions:

> Wolter's experience with postpartum depression is vastly more typical than Andrea Yates's. Indeed, PPD very rarely results in the kind of tragedy that unfolded in Houston last week. Still, it is a serious and

debilitating disorder that calls for prompt treatment. Unlike the "baby blues," a temporary period of weepiness that up to 80 percent of new mothers undergo, PPD is characterized by persistent feelings of anxiety, hopelessness and guilt, insomnia, lack of motivation and, sometimes, thoughts or fantasies of harming oneself—or even the baby. Doctors estimate that between 5 and 20 percent of all new mothers suffer from it. A much smaller number, about one woman in 1,000, experience the far more severe symptoms of postpartum psychosis, including hallucinations, paranoia and delusional, suicidal or homicidal thoughts. Like Yates, virtually all new mothers who harm their children are suffering from postpartum psychosis—not plain old PPD. "Every mom who's taking Prozac—or ought to be—is not going to smother her children and hang herself," says child psychiatrist Elizabeth Berger.[30]

Describing a continuum from the "baby blues" through postpartum depression and finally to postpartum psychosis, the article hedges its claims so as to cast doubt and suspicion on *all* mothers. While "normal" postpartum depression "rarely" results in tragedies such as Yates's infanticide, the possibility is not categorically denied. Women who suffer from postpartum depression, according to the article, sometimes do experience thoughts of harming themselves or their babies. Although "virtually all" mothers who harm their children are suffering from the more severe form of psychosis, the adjective "virtually" leaves room for some depressions to be homicidal without an escalated diagnosis. Similarly, Yates is presumed to be psychotic rather than just "plain old" depressed, but the first sentence of the excerpt places Yates and Wolter in parallel subject positions in relation to postpartum *depression*, not *psychosis*. Wolter's experiences with the illness—which does not include harming her children—is "more typical than" Yates's, but this phrasing suggests that Yates herself suffers from the same illness as Wolter. Yates is not definitively diagnosed within the text of the article; her presence serves as a cautionary tale to lend urgency to the description and identification of *all* depressed mothers as potentially dangerous.

The concluding statement from the child psychiatrist comments as much on the need for more diagnosis—and therefore more prescriptions for drugs such as Prozac—as it does on the likelihood that new mothers will harm their children. In the end, this paragraph exemplifies a trend toward sensational coverage that links forms of depression without clearly defining distinctions among them. The anxieties expressed by Danquah and Manning in their memoirs can be read as a natural result of such imprecision. If motherhood is constructed as always potentially homicidal, then all women of childbearing age become potential targets for intervention and careful monitoring.

The Ambiguous Logic of Not-Statements

The boundaries of depression remain invisible, in part, because depression appears to resemble "normal" affective states. In the *Handbook of Depression and Anxiety*, William Frosch introduces the text by writing,

> Depression and anxiety, both externally experienced and internally perceived, are part of the normal human repertoire of response to stress. In my opinion, those who never experience such feelings are seriously ill, unable to recognize or respond appropriately to the importance of danger and loss. On the other hand, the capacity to tolerate a 'normal expectable' level of each is a sign of mental health. Unfortunately, however, many of us are unable to withstand the impact of the usual vicissitudes of life and are overwhelmed by excessive stress or chronic strain.[31]

The "usual vicissitudes of life" shade into depression *only* when the individual cannot "withstand" them, but Frosch does not establish any reliable thresholds. In fact, he indicts "many of us" as potentially ill, if we are not resilient enough to cope with the stress and strain of life. As a gesture of sympathy, the linking of depression to everyday experiences is an inclusive one. In Danquah's words: "We have all, to some degree, experienced days of depression. Days when nothing is going our way, when even the most trivial events can trigger tears, when all we want to do is crawl into a hole and ask 'Why me?'"[32] Yet, as sympathetic as such comparisons may be, they nevertheless confuse the boundaries of illness, and this confusion leads to both over and underdiagnosis by individuals themselves and by their friends and relatives.

Much of depression's definition comes in the form of negation rather than affirmation of a precise illness. Such "not-statements" help distinguish between entities, but only in a relational and not an absolute fashion.[33] Further, not-statements form a link, albeit an oppositional one, between normal and abnormal states. In a categorical world, depression is *not* an extension of "normal emotions," it is a distinct entity. Wolpert hints at this view, suggesting that "even if there is a continuum, severe depression is an experience that bears little resemblance to mild depression."[34] Nevertheless, his stance admits "resemblance" between mild and severe forms of illness. A categorical stance, represented primarily by proponents of a biochemical model, might go further, labeling depression a brain disease, as one *Blues Buster* article does when it asserts: "Depression is not in your head. It's in your brain."[35] But, as Andrew Solomon points out, denying a continuum between sadness and depression flattens the illness experience and denies validity to a range of depressive identities: "This is perhaps the most alarming thing about current wisdom on depression: it dismisses the idea of a continuum and posits that a patient either has or doesn't have depression, is or is not depressed, as though to be a little bit depressed were the same as being a little bit pregnant. . . . Depression the illness is an excess of something common, not the introduction of something exotic."[36] For Solomon, and many others' commonsensical notions of depression, the continuum provides an important underlying cognitive structure that anchors depression alongside everyday emotional experiences.[37] Solomon's primary argument—that depression is "an excess of something common"—works to blur categorical thresholds, offering only quantity as an imprecise measure of illness.

In my corpus, such differentiation statements repeatedly tie the illness to sadness syntactically. Within such statements, a variety of negative stereotypes about sufferers gain voice and serve as further incentives for self-monitoring. In one advice column, Michael Yapko asserts that "depression is not a character defect, a weakness, a shameful condition, a disease that you caught somehow, or a curse from God. It is a hook in the stream of life that anyone can get snagged on under certain circumstances."[38] Yapko's first sentence repeats a series of pejorative characterizations about sufferers from depression in order to refute them. Nevertheless, the repetition of these stereotypes serves to confirm their cultural salience: even as they are denied, they are (re)voiced. Such negative characterizations are not replaced by positive terms for sufferers in Yapko's formulation, they are neutralized and deanimated by being described as mere "hooks" or snags. Depression may not be a "character defect," but it apparently catches individuals "under certain [unspecified] circumstances." Yapko attempts to universalize the illness but leaves only negative space where a definition might reasonably be expected.

In a similar encompassing move, one *Newsweek* article describes major depression as differing from common sadness primarily by degree. The article claims that "clinical depression is *more* than a low mood."[39] It makes this argument first by acknowledging that "feeling down is a common response to difficulty" and then by citing statistics that "as many as one in six people" will experience "Major Depression . . . at some time in their lives." The warrant and backing for this article's claim, however, are unstated, leaving the reader nothing but the sympathetic description of "common response[s]" to difficulties. Whether they are the character defects in Yapko's description, or negative life events in the *Newsweek* article, the only reference points for identifying depression in such not-statements are the same qualities that are being denied. In other words, even if the illness is not a character flaw or a response to bad news, it nevertheless exists in close relation to such attributes. The oppositional logic of such not-statements attempts to differentiate illness from everyday experience, but in doing so it locates the illness proximal to health and relies on "normal" sadness as a cognitive reference point.

One of the most common appositives for depression is the phrase "the blues." Although a lot of discursive energy is directed at differentiating the illness

TABLE 3.3

Headlines Linking Depression and "the Blues"

Headline

Having a Bad Hair Day of the Soul

Rhythm and the Blues

Online and Bummed Out

B6 Beats the Blues

The Baby Blues and Beyond

Singing End-of-Beach-Season Blues

Don't Let Your Baby Blues Go Code Red

Even CEOs Get the Blues

Five Years Old and Already Blue

SOURCE: Examples taken from research corpus of contemporary language about depression (1995–2005).

from the blues, the latter quite often serves as a synonym. Many kinds of depression are described using the common phrase: for example, the "baby blues" refers to postpartum depression, and the "winter blues" describes seasonal affective disorder (a cyclical depression tied to the seasons). Headlines are a key culprit in maintaining the definitional ambiguity wherein depression both *is* and *is not* "the blues" (see table 3.3). In a variety of article titles, depression is universalized and also trivialized by its association with the blues or similar colloquialisms such as "having a bad hair day" and being "bummed out." These quips operate within the discourse as opposing forces to the categorical impulses of not-statements: they trivialize and normalize the illness. The discourse, while ostensibly differentiating depression from the blues, works simultaneously to ensure that the illness is understood *as* the blues. The opposing vectors of differentiating depression from and also aligning it with "the blues" cancel each other out only within individual illness identities that must traverse the definitions of depression selectively. Readers of the discourse become literate when they write themselves into the multiple conflicting identities prescribed for them.

Complications and Co-occurrences: Depression and Heart Disease

As an argument for parity, depression sometimes appears alongside more culturally accepted disease entities, such as heart disease. This syntax intends to transfer legitimacy and comprehensibility from a more well understood disease to depression. In my corpus, this correlation draws on superficial similarities—heart disease is understood as a collection of related health problems—and on the co-occurrence of the two illnesses. Other diseases alongside which depression appears in the discourse include diabetes, cancer, hypertension, and stroke. Proximity does not, unfortunately, provide clarity of definition, however. While the statement, "Just like other illnesses, such as heart disease, depression comes in different forms,"[40] offers the comfort of similarity, it also does little to help define either illness. In other comparisons, depression ranks second to heart disease in physical disability, which gives a measure to its severity but again fails to help clarify what the illness might comprise. For example: "Depression is, after heart disease, the most physically debilitating illness, and it's progressive. You can't afford it."[41] In fact, depression's appearance alongside heart disease does more to confuse its boundaries than it does to legitimize it as a disease.

Discerning depression in cases of co-occurence becomes complicated because it may be the result of a primary illness or of a medication prescribed to treat another illness. In one article, we learn that "it may be difficult to discern a co-occurring depressive disorder in patients who present with other illnesses, such as heart disease, stroke, or cancer, which may cause depressive symptoms or may be treated with medications that have side effects that cause depression."[42] Here, depression may not fundamentally be real; it may be a mere side effect. In another instance, the interrelationship between depression and heart disease creates an additional urgency for diagnosis—depression can exacerbate the other illness: "What's more, it's become clear over the past several years that depression and heart disease don't just frequently co-exist, each leads to the other. Depression makes existing heart disease especially deadly; it also actually spurs the development of coronary artery disease."[43] Here, again, assertions of coexistence and causality do very little to help define depression or enable diagnosis. These associations succeed in making depression appear dangerous, but they obscure more than clarify its boundaries; they do not operate as analogies for illness, but rather as precipitators of (self) diagnosis. Within the discourse of depression, lexical, syntactic, and rhetorical structures all increase rather than decrease the definitional imprecision surrounding the illness, and this serves as a catalyst and a resource for practices of self-doctoring.

Describing depression in relation to diseases that seem to parallel it works, counterintuitively, to further confuse the contours of the illness. As in the cases of modifiers and notstatements, analogies with heart disease operate primarily to reinforce the ambiguities and risks associated with depression, without offering much clarity in terms of the exact relationship between the entities. The discourse of depression maintains an imprecise definition of depression that obligates individuals, particularly women, to read themselves into the illness in order to avoid the potential dangers, including complicating other co-morbid conditions, of remaining undiagnosed.

Translating Statistical into Personal Risk

Enhancing the imprecision of depression's definition, an expansive rhetoric of risk—including epidemiological figures and estimates of the economic and cultural impact of the illness—encourages more individuals to see themselves as ill. A series of statistics and estimates populates the discourse of depression, for example, the NIMH assertion that "in any given 1-year period, 9.5 percent of the population, or about 20.9 million American adults suffer from a depressive illness."[44] Such figures work to persuade readers of the *possibility* of their own inclusion in the "at risk" population. Further, recurrent calculations of lost work and diminished productivity as a result of depression compel self-identification with illness in order to remain with the "free market" economy.[45] In addition to the "economic cost" of depression,[46] and its associated health risks, which "you can't afford,"[47] recovery (often via pharmaceutical intervention) is signaled by statements such as, "Now *back at work*—and back to her old self she wishes she had started taking it [Paxil] earlier."[48] In this article, the woman's "old self" is predicated on her presence at work; her regret at not having taken medication earlier introduces an emotional appeal (pathos) to readers who may be risking their own employment by not treating their illnesses. The woman serves as a mouthpiece for the biochemical discourse, and her personal experience encourages others to identify themselves within that model for the sake of a productive economy. Assimilating generic "risk" of illness into individual identities proves to be one of the most coercive definitional moves of the discourse.

According to Carolyn Miller, "risk analysis" is one of the legacies of the U.S. civilian nuclear power enterprise.[49] Government support beginning in the late 1970s established what has become the "standard account" of risk analysis, an account that has privileged the expertise of risk *assessment* over the political processes of risk *management*. This privileging has resulted in a perceived separation of risk analysis from risk communication, "a false distinction" because, fundamentally, "risk analysis *is* a form of communicating about risk."[50] Further, Miller argues, the "substitution of expertise for ethos" in the discourse of risk analysis results in a loss of personal connection. An emphasis on expertise draws legitimacy from "narrow technical knowledge" and fails to draw from "moral values or goodwill or even practical judgment."[51] In the discourse of depression, expertise resides in the collection of demographic and lifetime risk figures, which remain dehumanized until they are either incorporated into vignettes within the discourse or adopted as self-definitional by readers via practices of self-doctoring.

Postindustrial economies, according to Ulrich Beck, constitute a "risk society" that is characterized by the "cultural blindness of daily life."[52] This blindness—stemming perhaps from the alienation of expertise from ethos—leads to apathy and a lack of political action. Worse, the "calculus of risks . . . promise[s] the impossible: events that have not yet occurred become the object of current action—prevention, compensation or precautionary after-care."[53] For the discourse of depression, this subjection of "events that have not yet occurred" to "current action" results in practices such as Kramer's "cosmetic psychopharmacology" and what one of the mental health professionals I interviewed describes as the "almost prophylactic" distribution of SSRI medications after the terrorist attacks of September 11, 2001. Yet, for Beck, there is hope to be found in the fact that "culture 'sees' in symbols."[54] The promise of "symbols" lies in their availability for rhetorical analysis. For example, in my interview with the mental health professionals, Laurie describes a documentary on electroconvulsive therapy (ECT). She applauds the documentary for "show[ing] like six months in [the woman's] life, leading up to her . . . getting ECT. Just [showing] how she had been out playing and laughing with her children, and then the next day just not even being able to get out of bed." What is important to Laurie, and for the possibility of self-care, is the fact that the documentary reveals so much of the woman's *life*. Encouraging individuals to place their illness experiences within the full context of their *lives* is an important first step toward a fully dialogical and rhetorical care of the self.

Such self-care, however, appears underdeveloped at best in the current discourse, which links *ethos* to epidemiology, catalyzing public action primarily within narrow biomedical parameters. Wolpert's case for the broad social impact of depression urges a current response to future (potential) illnesses: "The percentage of the population that will have a major depressive episode during their lifetime is about 10 percent though some studies have found rates around 15 percent. The largest study in the USA found that the chance of someone having a major depression during their lifetime is about one in six. The percentage of the population either experiencing depression or being in close contact with a depressed individual is thus frighteningly large."[55] Here, the logical appeal of concrete percentages gives way to an emotional appeal, suggesting that a "frighteningly large" proportion of the population is currently affected by depression. Further, his switch to present tense, from his earlier future predictions, indicates the immediate applicability of his findings. Responses to these findings, however, focus narrowly on the supposed biological causes of and treatments for depression. By contrast, Wolpert also wonders whether "public education about depression might provide an important way forwards." He concludes that "the only way to find out is to try it and see."[56] Education remains an apparently untried (and untested within contemporary research models) response to depression, but it offers a counterweight to strictly pharmaceutical responses to the illness.

A nuanced and, indeed, *rhetorical* education might examine the ubiquitous statistic that women are approximately twice as likely to be depressed as men (see table 3.4). As a piece of expert knowledge, this "fact" circulates within the discourse and serves as a primary influence on professional and self-assessments of what constitutes or defines depression. Indeed, as Linda Blum and Nena Stracuzzi point out, "Mental illness is not only gendered in biomedical terms, with disproportionate cases of particular disorders among male or female individuals; mental illness is also constructed and understood in terms that convey femininity or masculinity, that produce and police their boundaries."[57] The particularly discursive construction of gendered identities is

---

TABLE 3.4

Statements of Women's versus Men's Risk of Depression

Risk statement

By official counts, women in this country become depressed at nearly twice the rate (12 percent each year) as men (7 percent).

That incidence is twice the rate for the general population: one in 10 men and one in four women will have a clinical depressive episode in their lifetimes.

Girls, once they reach puberty, are twice as likely as boys to become depressed.

No matter how the numbers are counted, women are twice as likely as men to be diagnosed with unipolar major depression: 21.3% of women and 12.7% of men experience at least one bout of major depression over the course of their lifetime.

Unfortunately, women can get stuck in negative emotions, caught in a downward spiral of hopelessness and immobility. And that, she finds, is a major reason women are twice as likely to develop depression as men are.

Women experience depression about twice as often as men.

Depression can strike anyone regardless of age, ethnic background, socioeconomic status, or gender; however, large scale research studies have found that depression is about twice as common in women as in men.

Depression is a pervasive and impairing illness that affects both women and men, but women experience depression at roughly twice the rate of men.

Source: Examples taken from research corpus of contemporary language about depression (1995–2005).

an important determinant of who is labeled "mentally ill," and a significant portion of the discursive construction derives from expert statistics such as the one that shows a greater occurrence of depression in women than in men.

Table 3.4 documents, however, that this statistic takes many rhetorical forms. Citing "official counts," one source claims that women *become depressed* at twice the rate of men;[58] another uses the statistic to suggest that women are twice as likely *to be diagnosed* with depression;[59] a third claims that women *experience* depression twice as often.[60] Clearly, there are semantic differences among these three constructions: being *diagnosed* with an illness is not necessarily congruent with *experiencing* it. The convenience of the figure—twice as likely—seems to override questions of precision when accounting for the occurrences of the illness. The rhetorical effect of such imprecision, again, is to reach the broadest possible audience, in this case, women. For men, the repetition of this statistic clearly feminizes the illness and makes the underreporting of symptoms more likely. Men, whose risk appears to be merely *half* that of women (by any of the measures above), might fail to recognize themselves within these statistics at all. For both men and women, critical reading strategies—asking questions of data as "loose" as these—become important tactics for self-care. That one is "twice" or even "half" as likely to experience depression, in the end, does very little to define or delimit the experience of illness.

For men's illness identities, the feminizing effect of statistics such as those included in table 3.4 necessitates various hypermasculine rhetorical responses. Descriptions of male depression are often tied to unquestionably masculine identities such as athletes and successful businessmen. Men are encouraged to "confront" and "beat" their depression, and, if they are "brave enough," they can restore their masculinity in the process. Terry Bradshaw represents an ideal masculinity in one article: "Not every man can win a Super Bowl, but most can beat depression if they're brave enough to seek help. . . . Confronting depression is not about admitting weakness or defeat. More often, it's about restoring your mojo and reclaiming simple pleasures. Bradshaw, when asked what he enjoys now that his depression is treated, told me, 'Eatin' peanuts.' Now that's manhood."[61] The experience of depression, for Bradshaw, is a battle against depression *and* against the "negative typecasting" of men who suffer from it. Here, the "negative typecasting" derives primarily from the association of depression with women. "Manliness," the article asserts, "is tied up with strength, independence, efficiency and selfcontrol. Denying depression may help us [men] feign those virtues, but the cost of denial is huge."[62] The construction of a hypermasculine identity—emphasizing "restoring . . . mojo" and, even, "eatin' peanuts"—fails to offer men identities or rhetorical strategies to accommodate an illness that is not simply a matter of "muscle." Indeed, this and other articles work to maintain gendered social performances, particularly in statements such as: "Getting help with depression is as consistent with masculine ambitions as an exercise program or a solid financial plan."[63] Such statements help construct not only the available subjectivities for men suffering from depression, but also those available for healthy men, who ought to aspire to exercise programs and solid financial planning.

The feminization of depression represents a particularly thorny problem for diagnostic reliability. At one point in our interview, Laurie (the clinical psychologist) refers to depression as a "woman's disease." I ask for clarification:

KE: Laurie, you said earlier, as sort of an aside, [that] depression is a woman's disease?

LAURIE: Mmm hmm.

KE: Why?

LAURIE: Two to, three to one. Two to one. Two to one; three to one. One way or the other.

OTHERS: [overlapping] Two to one.

LAURIE: Yeah, I was going to say that it depends on age groupings and things like that, but it's just, you know, mine [i.e., clients] are all women. You [to Ellen] said that you predominantly saw, what, 80 percent women? I think we see women that are depressed, and . . . we see men who are depressed, but they don't generally get there first. I was thinking of all the perpetrators I see. . . . *None* of them have a depression diagnosis, until they've been in perpetrator treatment for a while, and you start stripping away the anger, and you start finding out where that anger came from, and then you just rip off this sort of façade, and you see this incredible amount of depression. But, it's buried deep, and the first thing you see is they're violent, so they come up with anger management and all sorts of things like that, which are not really very good treatments any more, we know.

In response to my request for clarification, Laurie and her colleagues cite the statistical evidence for women's greater risk for depression. The accuracy of the statistic seems only secondary: Laurie suggests that "one way or the other" the statistic is adequate proof of her statement that depression is a woman's disease. The generalized statistic is supported by the mental health professionals' own clinical experiences. As they continue to talk, however, they begin to deconstruct the statistic and search for additional explanations. Ellen, the psychiatrist, picks up after Laurie's last turn:

ELLEN: Well, I think there's also a reason that women may have more depression. And, I think that it's societal. As women, I think we are still frequently trapped into roles of being helpless, or we're expected to be helpless, and I think that that's a real setup for somebody becoming depressed.

OTHERS: Mmm hmm.

JOAN: I wonder, too, how much of the two-to-one has to do with what you were talking about, like the fact that [you] don't see men coming saying, "I'm feeling depressed." I wonder how much of it is sort of like, or how much we're tuned to not

LAURIE: [overlapping] looking for it I mean that gets back to your suggestion about the bias. How much we're really not looking for depression in men, because when we first see men—at least for me the first thing that triggers is not depression. I start with a sort of my wide net and go down. When I see women the first thing I do is start with depression and go out.

Ellen focuses on social conditioning, which may contribute to women's vulnerability, but Joan begins to make the rhetorician's argument. She wonders whether the statistic might be influenced by men's rhetorical performances (or their lack of particular self-diagnostic practices). In response, Laurie's admission that with women in her clinical practices, "the first thing [she does] is start with depression," demonstrates the material effects of the discourse. Even experts find themselves responding to individuals in prescribed ways based not on immediate presentation but on the expectation modeled within the discourse. It is ultimately unimportant whether women are twice or three times as likely as men to be depressed. That they are *more* likely is enough to shape clinical and individual performances. Importantly, Laurie's statement suggests that depression is central, at the core of an individual's experiences. Beliefs such as this make depression more than an illness; they make it an identity. The confusion and ultimate disregard of the statistics is also telling. It recalls Susan Nolen-Hoeksema's assertion that "no matter how you define depression, after puberty women show more depression than men."[64] The mythic quality of these numbers serves as a foundation for other social and cultural responses to depression.

Starting with depression and "going outward," Laurie's practices also situate depression at the very center of women's identities. This makes it more than an illness; depression is a (gendered) identity. Within my corpus, a variety of compounds with *self-* associate the illness with critical attention to individual identities. Table 3.5 displays the variety of such compounds, many of which indicate largely negative attention to the self. Phrases such as *self-destruction* and *self-harm* focus on the deleterious effects of the illness, but phrases such as *self-aggrandizing, self-deprecating*, and *self-obsessed* suggest judgment and social disapproval of the ill self. Additionally, many of the compounds draw attention to practices of self-monitoring (e.g., *self-appraisal, self-assessment, self-aware, self-management*) that represent the process of submitting the self to treatment regimes and medical institutions. Importantly, these compounds and other references to the self come to rest within women's health and illness identities. Wurtzel describes herself as having a "morose character," her depression as

TABLE 3.5

Compounds with *Self-* in the Corpus

Compound	No.	Compound	No.	Compound	No.
Esteem	47	Cure	3	Control	2
Medication	7	Focus	3	Correct	2
Worth	7	Harm	3	Deprecating	2
Destruction	6	Image	3	Diagnosed	2
Help	6	Inflicted	3	Fulfilling	2
Critical	5	Injurious	3	Guardianship	2
Pity	5	Management	3	Hypnosis	2
Appraisal	4	Aggrandizing	2	Obsessed	2
Assessment	4	Aware	2	Soothing	2
Welfare	4	Censorship	2	Talk	2
Conscious	3				

SOURCE: Examples taken from research corpus of contemporary language about depression (1995–2005).

"everything about me. It colored every aspect of me so thoroughly, and I became resigned to that."[65] For Wurtzel, her depression is rooted in her "character"; she is inextricable from it. In effect, she has lost her self to the illness. Manning, herself a psychologist, describes the medical equivalent of this phenomenon, where depression becomes a patient's whole identity rather than a separate, transient experience. She writes, "In the midst of discussing cases with several colleagues, someone refers to a patient as 'a thirty-five-year-old manic depressive.' I cringe, mentally leave the case discussion, and retreat into my own head. . . . I think about the difference between *having* something and *being* something. They are only words, but I'm struck by how much they convey about the manner in which the shorthand of mental illness reduces the essence of people in ways that labels for other serious illnesses do not."[66] The power of diagnostic labels to supersede individual identities resonates most definitely for women, who are described as at greater risk for depression.

The women who spoke with me about their own symptoms of depression—and it is important that none of these women were at the time diagnosed with depression or even experiencing a level of symptoms that would qualify them for diagnosis—seemed to have great difficulty separating their symptoms from their self-assessments. In one group, Claire responds to my question asking for a definition of depression:

CLAIRE: Well, I would say it's when you're sad. I know people because of circumstances in their life can get sad for a few months and then it goes away after. So, to me depression is more than just being sad for, you know, two months or something. It's something that carries on and it affects your daily life. It affects your motivation, your energy, and maybe you're extra emotional and you cry even more, and that's what it means to me.

PAIGE: Can I ask you a question? Sorry. You said earlier that you were, that you feel like you're an overemotional person. Do you think that's your nature? Or do you think that's a stage that you're in, because you feel depressed now or what?

Paige asks Claire to define *herself* rather than her feelings of depression. Wondering if Claire's sadness might just be her "nature" as an "overemotional person," Paige gives voice to the primary product of depression's definitional imprecision for women, namely, a strong suspicion of the self and its experiences. The women attempt to frame their experiences, but they do so by making use of the resources of the discourse of depression, which statistically constructs them as twice as likely to be depressed. In such a rhetorical environment, even normal emotions become subject to scrutiny and potential diagnosis.

In my corpus, *depression* remains an ambiguous and widely applied label for a variety of populations, experiences, and activities. This constitutive imprecision reinforces individuals' practices of self-doctoring and, particularly, their suspicious orientations toward gendered illness identities. Both men and women are subject to these discursive pressures, which force men to perform hypermasculine identities in order to receive treatment, on the one hand, and which subject women's core identities to illness labels, on the other. Depression remains intimately connected to notions of the self for women, and as such it inspires self-questioning and self-monitoring. For example, one of the women I interviewed describes how she came to hear of my research interviews:

MEI: Um, well, I saw it [the flyer] in the campus center. I was actually waiting for the bus [laughs]. I didn't have anything to do, so I read the bulletin board. And then, oh, I think it was because it's—I think depression is kind of interest[ing]. It's a fascinating area because it affects so many people, but I really don't know what it is. And, I don't know if I have it or [not], but I do know that there's some feelings that I wonder if they are depression or not. And so, I sent you an email to see what it was about.

Mei's story gives evidence for the growth of self-doctoring practices—attending a research interview on "language and depression" must be considered such a practice—out of the imprecision of depression's definition. Mei admits that she finds depression "interesting" and "fascinating," but also that she doesn't "really know what it is." Her transition from considering depression as an illness that "affects so many people" to her own self-assessment of "I don't know whether I have it" suggests that she has taken up the recruitment flyer, in part, as a definition both of the illness and of herself. Despite the fact that the word *depression* appears only in the title of the study and not in the criteria for inclusion listed, Mei has nevertheless read the flyer as a definition of illness and has agreed to talk with me, in part, to satisfy her curiosity about her own potential identity as a depression sufferer. Her description of how she came to contact me distills the major persuasive moves in the discourse of depression: an imprecise definition invites questioning, self-assessment follows, and self-diagnosis looms as the potential result.

Practices of definition typically promote clarity and mark boundaries. Within the discourse of depression, however, definitional moves fail to promote this sort of precision. Instead, categorical labels, adjectival modifications, not-statements, and analogies all sustain porous boundaries, a move that encourages practices of self-questioning and self-doctoring. While the mental health professionals I interviewed seem to support a more personalized articulation of depression in their therapeutic interventions, they nevertheless proved susceptible to gendered assumptions about the illness. The discourse of depression fosters a strategically imprecise definition in order to expand the potential patient population and to encourage practices of self-doctoring. Operating within the discourse, individuals and health-care experts have a limited range of tactical responses. Nevertheless, one such potential response lies in figurative descriptions; metaphors for depression evoke more contextualized definitions and serve as a possible avenue for promoting a critical rhetorical orientation toward the discourse.

4

Isolating Words

Metaphors That Shape Depression's Identities

The apparently straightforward algebra of depression might be expressed by the following equations: Depression = X; X ≠ "the blues"; X > normal sadness. But, as the variety of imprecise definitional practices reveal, the problem of X remains. Or, perhaps more accurately, the problem if X is multiplied within the discourse as the result of strategies that implicate a broad range of experiences as potential illness. When equations fail, metaphoric and figurative language often provides an alternative mode of explanation: Tracy Thompson calls her depression, simply, "The Beast"; a synaesthetic transfer from feeling to vision underwrites references to depression as "the blues" and "darkness"; and classical mythologies credit Saturn with influence over melancholia.[1] The figurative resources of the English language provide new avenues for expression, but within my sample of contemporary discourse, the metaphoric definitions of depression depict the illness in largely isolated, individual settings. This pattern reiterates the discourse's emphasis on personal responsibility for self-doctoring and masks other potential relationships, particularly social and community-based responses to the illness. Broad categories of metaphoric expression—animal, geographical, mechanical, and communicative—populate the discourse with images that return compulsively to the self.

Rhetorically, metaphors help define through transference: qualities of a known source are attributed to an unknown target, thereby translating the unknown into terms that enable communication in at least two senses. First, on a pragmatic level, metaphors deliver *messages*, in this case definitions of an otherwise indescribable illness experience. In addition, however, metaphors promise to transfer *experiences* from one individual to another; they create points of human contact, which invoke empathy and identification. In both cases, metaphors appear to promise connection, yet within the discourse of

depression the most common metaphors offer only the recognition and reitera-
tion of isolation.

Literal language is often accused of being inadequate for the purpose of
true communication, opening a space for metaphoric translations. In his
comprehensive history of depression, Stanley Jackson asserts that "there is no
literal statement that would convey to a reader the distress of being in the
throes of a severe depression. Without knowing from firsthand experience or
having at least learned with empathy directly from the distressed eloquence of
a sufferer, it would require the enhancement of a metaphorical expression
to bridge the gap of understanding, to draw the reader at least vicariously
into the troubling subjective world of such a sufferer."[2] Jackson's conclusion
illuminates the power of metaphoric constructions to "bridge the gap of understanding" between healthy and ill individuals. Metaphors work to produce what
literal language cannot: comprehension and also, crucially, experience in those
who do not suffer from depression. They imply a transportation across conceptual boundaries that is both necessary (for the depressed individual) and
alluring (for the healthy). Jackson writes that metaphorical expression not only
bridges the gap—his own metaphor implying the topographic separation
between the healthy and the ill—but it also *draws the reader* across that bound-
ary and into a new subjectivity. As a consequence of empathy and of
metaphoric transference, healthy individuals risk being drawn into the illness
experience themselves. While they remain outsiders, their vicarious experiences with depression—via metaphor—locate them on the border between
health and illness. And, while that border is often presumed impervious to
literal description, the figurative language surrounding depression invites
identification with the illness and therefore also an intensified scrutiny of the
geographies of the self.

Exploring the contours of depression through the metaphors that describe
it reveals much about contemporary practices of self-doctoring. The importance of sympathetic communication, for example, suggests a desire for social
connection even in the throes of an illness characterized by *dis*connection. The
structure and content of metaphors for depression, however, reinforce the isolation of individuals and postpone the possibility of social connection until
health is resumed. In fact, contemporary metaphors within the discourse of
depression reinforce the work of biological psychiatry, narrowing the experience of depression to the neurochemical processes in an individual's brain.
Social networks play only ancillary roles in these metaphors, and when they
appear, they do so as symptoms or as potential victims of the individual's
depression. These metaphoric and figurative descriptions of depression shape
illness identities, isolating individuals within their physical bodies and making
them responsible for returning themselves to health.

Metaphoric language structures both sufferers' experiences of illness and also the social, institutional, and medical responses to it. What begins as an imprecise description can become an organizing principle in medical practice and self-doctoring. Descriptors such as *darkness* and feeling *weighted down* have been repeated so often and for so long that they have ceased to be recognized as metaphorical at all.[3] This transfer—from an approximation (metaphor) to a fact—carries important scientific and ethical implications. Early modern humoral theory asserted that black bile and vapors arising from the spleen literally blackened the mind and spirit.[4] The figurative alignment of depression with blackness continues to produce illness identities that remain "in the dark" and impenetrable to the "light" of investigation. Further, it complicates non-white illness identities, because those individuals cannot posit their healthy selves in opposition to the darkness of depression.[5] Cultural assumptions, particularly within and about the African American community, limit the ability to recognize depression in people of color. While this cannot be blamed entirely on the figurative construction of depression as specifically *black*, such cultural blindness certainly receives rhetorical support from the discourse.

For scientific engagements with the illness, the literalization of figurative language—as in the early modern assumption that brains were literally blackened by depression—has the potential to direct resources and research. For individuals, metaphoric and figurative expressions may manifest physically within the body. For example, the metaphorical notion of a mind "weighted down" in the early English language eventually took on the form of a physical sensation: heavy limbs. And, by the ninth century, the term *heavy* reflected this transition acquiring depressive symptomology—"oppressed condition of the body, members, or senses; torpor; drowsiness; dullness; want of animation"—among its meanings.[6] In seventeenth- and eighteenth-century scientific thought, fluid flow theories asserted that blood had "slowed down" in depressed individuals, leading to the use of such phrases to describe the experience of the illness. As these theories fell out of favor in the nineteenth century, so did the use of this figurative construction of depression. Yet both fluid-flow and humoral notions have endured, surviving today in depression's symptomology, for example, in the *DSM* criterion of "psychomotor retardation" (being slowed down) and in the prevailing understanding of an imbalance of chemicals as the root cause of depression (perhaps substituting chemical balances for humoral ones).

Figurative ways of explaining an emotional state may eventually come to serve as literal explanations for the disorder; they begin to manifest in physical symptoms. Metaphors describe and also structure our behavior in the world. Canonical work on cognitive metaphors demonstrates, for example, that orientational metaphors such as UP IS GOOD and DOWN IS BAD are rooted in the realities of corporeal activity.[7] As such, they become deep cognitive structures capable of generating additional metaphors, for example the understanding of depression as "being down" or as "falling into an abyss," both of which rely for their comprehension on the conceptual equation DOWN IS BAD. Additionally, the equation implies its opposite, so remedies for depression promise to "lift" spirits, "boost" morale, or simply keep one on higher ground, safe from going "over the edge."

Beyond the linguistic productivity of metaphors, such figurative understandings of reality have the power to shape the direction of future research. For example, biology textbooks and other cultural artifacts from the 1970s often used the gendered roles of traditional fairy tales as a trope to describe the process of fertilization.[8] Characterizing sperm as active and valiant—venturing into hostile territory, vying for the prize of the passive egg—texts such as these encourage research questions that view the potential activities of each cell according to expected roles.[9] In the case of depression, similar ontological effects occur, most obviously within the framework that postulates an imbalance of the neurotransmitter serotonin as the cause of depression. As a consequence of this formulation, individuals come to expect both an ideal balance of serotonin to exist and methods of measuring and maintaining that balance to be the singular solution to depression. Further, research funding and project resources in the scientific community flow toward neurobiology as a result of this foundational understanding of the illness.

When access to depression is available largely through figurative language, that language ironically threatens to foreclose creative thinking and alternative solutions. Andrew Solomon refers to this phenomenon using his own imagery of the disconnection of language from action: "Perhaps depression can best be described as emotional pain that forces itself on us against our will, and then breaks free of its externals . . . It is tumbleweed distress that thrives on thin air, growing despite its detachment from the nourishing earth. It can be described only in metaphor and allegory."[10] For Solomon, "linguistic vagary" is both intrinsic to depression—which "can be described only in metaphor"—and a socially constructed phenomenon of the late twentieth century. The loss of connection with "the nourishing earth" that characterizes the "distress" of depression is, to some extent, the loss of the distinction between metaphoric source and target. As metaphor and analogy become the *only* tools with which to understand depression, the rhetoric becomes the reality of experience—both for sufferers, who come to understand their *selves* through the language of the illness, and for researchers, who have access to the illness only through that language. In each of the broad categories of figurative expression within my sample of contemporary public texts about depression, the self becomes increasingly isolated and responses to depression become restricted to matters of chemistry or of individual self-help. As such, the metaphors for depression encourage narrow practices of self-doctoring that fail to participate in social, community, or other dialogical responses to the illness experience.

Battling the Beast Within

Given the twentieth century popularity of declaring war on entities from which we wish to extricate ourselves, it is perhaps surprising that depression has not been figured as an opponent of this sort. In fact, within my corpus, the word *war* appears only twenty-six times, and only once referring to "the war against mental illness."[11] Further, in this singular instance, the war targets both *illness* and *sufferers*, who are hard to distinguish from the actual enemy. The article, titled "Crisis on Campus," offers the following assessment of the rise in demand for mental health services on college campuses: "Today they [college counseling centers] are the newest front line in the war against mental illness, struggling to manage swarms of students with serious depression and anxiety disorders."[12] Forming a "front line" against "swarms of students," such centers seem to be battling both *mental illness* and the *students* themselves. As the frontier outposts, college counseling centers work to "manage" the overwhelming and disorganized masses of students who apparently need help. That *management* becomes a weapon in the war against mental illness further implies structural and bureaucratic responses rather than military ones. This single instance of a war on mental illness directs attention toward the students themselves, who must be accommodated, instead of toward the illness, its causes, or its potential cures (as we might expect from parallel constructions such as the "war on cancer").

Similar to this curious war on college campuses, the use of the terms *enemy* and *enemies* within my collection of texts demonstrates the congruity between the illness and individuals themselves. Table 4.1 provides a concordance list—providing several word contexts on either side of the term—for *enemy/enemies*. The list includes three references to the *illness* as an enemy and four to *people* as enemies. Of the three references to *depression* as an enemy, two occur in articles about soldiers and depression, arguably a topical field that would cue the term more readily than other scenarios. The third reference to depression as an enemy casts it as a "tractable" one, lessening its power to threaten and thereby diminishing the force of its implied battle. Conversely, the four references to *people* as enemies acknowledge adversarial relationships and direct aggression interpersonally rather than against illness. Janet Jackson's assertion that she and brother Michael are "not enemies in any way" suggests that they are nevertheless not close. More specifically, two references suggest that *enemies* help monitor the self, giving them a powerful position in relation to the individual. Finally, the "legal battle" fought by a father to allow his daughter, who was in a vegetative state, to die accrues enemies to him, signaling his increasing isolation and disconnection as he becomes more depressed. These references, far from declaring war on depression, cast depression *sufferers* as enemies whose experiences are antagonistic to community.

TABLE 4.1

Concordance for "Enemy/ies" in the Corpus

a disease that . . . has proven to be a tractable	enemy	From chronic, low-grade depression
because depression shouldn't be yet another	enemy	on the battlefield
Psychological problems, she says, are an	enemy	that no soldier should face alone
Ask not only your friends but also your	enemies	how much of an obsessor you are
rely on others—family, friends, even	enemies	–to give you accurate feedback
We're not	enemies	in any way
legal battle made news and	enemies	almost monthly

SOURCE: Examples taken from research corpus of contemporary language about depression (1995–2005).

In a similar way, the occurrences of the terms *battle, battles,* and *battled* emphasize the isolation and solitary nature of individuals' struggle with depression. Of twenty-five occurrences of the terms, three refer to wartime battles, and four more refer to legal battles, rather than engagements with the illness itself (table 4.2). The remaining references to "battling depression" include several explicit indicators of isolation, including "a battle she had to fight *on her own*";[13] "Mrs. Gore's *own* battle";[14] and "her *private* battle with clinical depression."[15] Battling depression does not always mean fighting the illness itself, rather it can also mean fighting for the self and its representation, as in "her mother's long battle with the stigma of her disease." In this instance, again, the battle turns inward. It is significant, though perhaps unsurprising, that these examples are predominantly female. The lexical field for battle would at first seem to suggest a masculine collocation. However, when the battle is understood as primarily internal and interpersonal, as is the case in the discourse of depression, the association with women becomes a manifestation of stereotypical assumptions about women's greater struggles with themselves.

Such internal, individual battles with illness do not conform to the promise of the military campaign. Full military units do not march into battle against depression; individuals and individual pharmaceutical agents do all of the fighting. In her memoir *Prozac Diary,* Lauren Slater describes Prozac in these terms: "It was a drug with the precision of a Scud missile, launched miles away from its target only to land, with a proud flare, right on the enemy's roof."[16] For Slater, the distance from which the assault is launched is as important as the precision of the strike. Her description emphasizes her isolation; indeed, it makes her a dangerous target for the "proud flare" of military attack.

This military and chemical fantasy—that a "surgical strike" is possible and desirable in times of war and in cases of depression—empties the illness of its social embedding. In order to launch a Prozac missile at one's brain, one must forget the other inhabitants (systems) that will be affected by the strike. A "clean" drug—one that appears to have very few side effects—is akin to a "surgical" military strike. Yet the definition of "clean" must be questioned in both cases. For antidepressants, the "low side-effect profile" of SSRI drugs nevertheless includes significant sexual dysfunctions for many, as Slater acknowledges in her memoir. The military metaphor implies that such collateral damage to one's sexual satisfaction is ultimately insignificant in the face of a successful strike against depression.[17] Within the discourse of depression, wartime images do not marshal troops or indicate allied forces; instead, they encourage individual and isolated engagements with the self, and, specifically, with neurochemical systems. The reality—the *battle*—of illness does not conform to the promise of the military campaign. Such references, therefore, further isolate individuals within their experiences of illness, suggesting to them that they are solitary fighters in a war that others have already won.

TABLE 4.2

Concordance for "Battle/s/d" in the Corpus

are many fronts on which to wage the	battle	against depression, there is a risk
This was a	battle	she had to fight on her own
	Battle	of the Sexes
can prolong the misery, resulting in a	battle	with depression that can last a
about her recent	battle	with a serious postpartum
dressed in full camouflage with two	battle	knives he'd been issued in Iraq.
Don't show the psychic wounds of	battle,	until after they're sent home.
over other Faxil patents. "They lost this	battle,	but the war's not over," said
58, who had a well-documented	battle	with mental illness
was a reference to Mrs. Gore's own	battle	with depression
more young men died of suicide than in	battle.	Though overall U.S. suicide rates
Her mother's long	battle	with the stigma of her disease
presidential campaign—and her private	battle	with clinical depression
Ironically, the court	battle	—the mission to win on his
"And then the highly public	battle	to 'win' the right to have his child
The wrenching legal	battle	made news and enemies almost
Kitty Dukakis chronicles	battle	with manic-depression and
Jamison first went public about her own	battles	with manic depression in 1995
"the men and women whose	battles	are the primary subject of this
Jack Nicholson's heroic McMurphy	battles	sadistic Nurse Ratchet on a
Two years later the court	battles	began with Jeffrey, who had
For the next year and a half, the two	battled	cultural myths and personal
risk for an Internet addiction, having	battled	alcohol and drug abuse and
Ms Rose, 31, who has	battled	crippling bouts of depression
a top executive who not only	battled	depression but is comfortable

SOURCE: Examples taken from research corpus of contemporary language about depression (1995–2005).

In alignment with these internal, private battles, bestial metaphors within the discourse of depression rarely evoke mythic or terrible beasts that must be battled and slain; more often it is the *self* at war. Manning writes of her fear of a future encounter with depression: "The terror of possible depression in the 'future' haunts me daily. I hate that dragon. It is my enemy. I am vigilant for it, scrambling to find out how I can prevent it from returning."[18] In this description, both the *terror* and the possible future *depression* are characterized as a "dragon" and as an "enemy." The terror she feels in anticipation of a future depression inspires constant vigilance from Manning, yet her fortifying activities engage with her current self rather than strictly with her possible future depression. In a similar personalizing gesture, Styron describes his father as having "battled the gorgon" of depression, but speaks of his own illness in far more intimate and familiar terms: "When it [depression] finally came to me, it was in fact no stranger, not even a visitor totally unannounced; it had been tapping at my door for decades."[19] The metaphoric beast of depression retains its menace, but as an abstraction; when it appears to individuals, it takes the form of an expected companion.

Jeffery Smith writes at the beginning of his memoir that "my familiar was stalking me again. I felt its breath on my neck hairs. I could smell it."[20] The sensual nature of this connection represents the intimacy of depression for its victims. Thompson's "beast" at first seems to retain the true animal—and outsider—status inherent in the metaphor. "I call him 'Beast' because it suits him," but she immediately qualifies this description. She writes, "I imagine 'him' not as a creature but as a force, something that has slipped outside the bounds of natural existence, a psychic freight train of roaring despair. For most of my life, the Beast has been my implacable and unpredictable enemy, disappearing for months or years, then returning in strength."[21] While Thompson denies the animal or human nature of her "beast," she nevertheless refers to it as "him" throughout her memoir. The gender of Thompson's beast reflects her memoir's consistent attention to her relationships with men, particularly to Thomas, a love who ultimately helps her confront her illness, but who also appears overbearing and critical at moments when Thompson herself is most vulnerable. Even as she casts "The Beast" as her enemy, Thompson cannot banish it (or Thomas himself) from her life. For both Smith and Thompson, then, depression is partially externalized through metaphoric beasts, but the intimate connections between self and beast ensure that the illness is never far from their consciousness of themselves.

The potential, inherent in bestial metaphors, to externalize depression resists the discursive alignment of self with illness, and thus appears to open a space for self-care as opposed to self-doctoring. However, these metaphors tend to settle in the domestic and familiar regions of the animal kingdom, suggesting that the illness ought to be domesticated rather than eradicated. In the

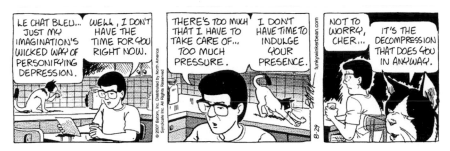

FIGURE 6. *Funky Winkerbean,* August 29, 2007. (*Funky Winkerbean* © Bantom. Inc. North American Syndicate)

summer of 2007, Lisa, a main character in Tom Batiuk's comic strip *Funky Winkerbean,* is dying of breast cancer. Visiting her grieving husband, *le chat bleu* serves as an externalization of emotions he cannot acknowledge (figure 6). In the first two panels of the August 29 strip, Les is seated at the kitchen table while the cat licks its paw and stretches on the counter behind him. Les explains the cat's presence as "just my imagination's wicked way of personifying depression." Claiming he is under "too much pressure . . . to indulge [the cat's/depression's] presence," Les does not look directly at the animal. In the final panel of the strip, *le chat bleu* and Les share a sidelong glance while the cat offers cold comfort: "Not to worry *cher* . . . It's the decompression that does you in anyway."

This comic offers a vivid reenactment of many popular assumptions about depression. It implies that feelings of grief such as those Les is experiencing are to be "indulged" (or not) by sufferers, thus casting depression as a *choice* rather than an illness. In addition, Les is alone in his kitchen, revealing and reenacting the isolation from families or social groups experienced by sufferers. This isolation—reinforced by other metaphoric constructions of the illness—entails a singular rather than a collective response to the illness. Les will have to confront *le chat bleu* himself, alone, after his wife passes away. Finally, the presence of a domestic animal as the metaphoric representation of depression suggests the intimacy (*cher* may be translated as "dear" from the French) and the familiarity of the illness, but this is revealed to be only partially accurate. Indeed, the striking contrast between the normal catlike behavior of *le chat bleu* in the first two frames, in which it appears in proper proportion to Les, and the final frame, in which its facial and verbal expressions are menacing, mirrors the complexity of depression itself. The illness, at once domesticated and an aberration, menaces from within the safety and isolation of one's home and one's self.

A depression information and research organization affiliated with the University of New South Wales in Australia calls itself "The Black Dog Institute." In its web logo, a human hand makes a shadow puppet figure of a dog; the hand's shadow, however, is that of a real dog's head, not the approximation made by a human hand. In this image, the utterly porous boundaries between the self, represented by the hand, and the disease, represented by the dog, illustrate the complexities of metaphoric representations of depression. This visual metaphor risks tautology: illness and the physical self are indistinguishable. While Winston Churchill is often credited with popularizing the term "black dog"—he did indeed refer to his own depression in this way—the linguistic record indicates that the term has a much longer, more vernacular history. Indeed, Churchill's use of the phrase draws on several centuries of nursery rhyme and folk history, as well as alludes to the literary and personal uses of "black dog" that date at least to the eighteenth century, when Samuel Johnson corresponded with Mrs. Thrale.

In the nineteenth century, popular fiction by Walter Scott and Robert Louis Stevenson recirculated the phrase. Churchill's use, however, has stuck in contemporary cultural memory as epitomizing stoic masculine resistance to illness. In use, the phrase "a black dog on your back" evokes both a literal attack (the dog having leaped onto your back) and the stalking of prey, both of which might be the familiar habit of hunting hounds, and of a particular form of masculinity. Yet the simplicity of the black dog domesticates the illness, making it a familiar (almost familial) companion. Similarly, in recent years, *New Yorker* writer Andrew Solomon has described his own depression as "slinking in on its little cat feet."[22] The choice of animal—whether black dog or (blue) cat—represents a metaphoric extension and externalization of the experience of depression. Nevertheless, these extensions remain extremely close to home and remain in the private spheres as much as possible. According to Solomon, "depression cannot be wiped out so long as we are creatures conscious of our own selves."[23] The illness inhabits the self so thoroughly that it becomes more companion than enemy.

The rhetorical force of metaphor lies in its ability to transfer qualities from the familiar term, the "source," to the less well understood term, its "target." Unlike its semantic cousin the simile, which explicitly maintains only the *similarity* between source and target, metaphor sets up a strong identification between its terms. When the semantic transfer is complete, the metaphor becomes reality, altering the physical and conceptual world. *Le chat bleu* is a personification of Les's depression—the illness come to life—rather than simply an imaginative representation of it. Tautology is a potential result of metaphor turned into reality. This possibility resides in what is often called a "dead metaphor," a literalization resulting from natural processes of language change. These dead metaphors also have the potential to obscure the workings of approximation and analogy in our thinking. In the case of metaphors for depression, the assimilation between source and target has implications for the available illness identities as well as for the conduct of research and treatment.

In Matthew Johnstone's self-help picture book, *Living with a Black Dog*, the visual constriction of metaphor into tautology manifests in several illustrations.

The Australian title of the book is *I Have a Black Dog* and the change from ownership (in the Australian title) to companionship (in the U.S. version) is suggestive of an intimate relationship between depression sufferers and their illnesses. Rather than a proprietary relationship—implied by *having* a black dog—the progressive tense of *living with* implies daily engagement. The text and the illustrations in the book align closely with the Australian title—much of this book is devoted to acknowledging the existence of the black dog, rather than to strategies for interacting with him. But in many of the illustrations, the collapse of protagonist and represented illness suggest a self fundamentally identified with and recognized by the illness.

On the cover of the book, the man sits on a bench and the shadow he casts takes the form of a black dog. The shape that the man takes in the world—the amount of sunlight his form obscures—is that of his figurative depression. In another striking image within the text, the man crouches on all fours, and superimposed on him, completely encompassing him, is the shadow of the black dog. In yet another image, the man looks into his bathroom mirror and sees not his own face reflected but the face of the black dog (figure 7). Here the metaphorical dog becomes not a possession (I *have* a black dog) but an identity (I *am* a black dog). The text accompanying this image—"A Black Dog can surprise

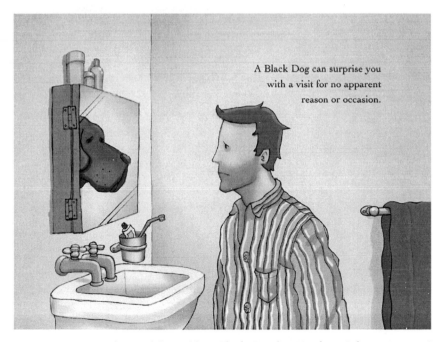

FIGURE 7. Image from *Living with a Black Dog* by Matthew Johnstone 2006. (Reproduced by arrangement with the copyright holder, Matthew Johnstone, 2009)

you, with a visit for no apparent reason or occasion"—seems to imply that the reflection is merely a *visitor* rather than an identity, but the image depends on the man seeing himself in the mirror *as* his illness. He must understand himself to be the (unwelcome) visitor in order to accept the responsibility of living with his depression. Thus, metaphoric creatures offer companionship and potential externalization of illness, but they also risk an intimacy that identifies *selves* with depression.

Such animal familiars may, perhaps, offer themselves as guides toward more tactics of self-care. Indeed, Johnstone's book is a model of this sort of engagement with the illness. Instead of threatening dragons and monsters, such domestic pets suggest resilience rather than dominance. In one issue of the *Blues Buster Newsletter*, parents write to Michael Yapko for help with their five-year-old daughter who is suffering from depression. They refer to her illness as a "sadness monster," but Yapko suggests alternative tactics: "On one level, calling [your daughter's] feelings the 'sadness monster' seems a supportive strategy. On a deeper level, though, she is learning that her feelings are enduring and formidable—even parts of her to be feared because they are 'monstrous.' Her emotions now have form and substance, a life all their own, which may prevent her from learning how to cope with them. She is being unintentionally reinforced for expressing and succumbing to her fears, rather than learning how to manage and transcend them. Start talking to her instead about how her feelings are a part of her but not all of her; they vary, they are potentially useful as teachers, and they can't completely define her."[24] Even at this girl's extremely young age, Yapko advocates that feelings of fear and anxiety be assimilated within her self-comprehension: they should become "a part of" her, "manage[d] and transcend[ed]" but nevertheless internalized. Indeed, the connection between depression and the self is often characterized in the terms of an intimate relationship or romance. Styron speaks of his "involvement with the illness," suggesting not simply a battle or encounter, but a long-term and multifaceted, interpersonal engagement.[25] The danger of this intimacy, of course, is the danger of the man in Johnstone's illustration viewing himself *as* his depression. Its potential, however, is a more complex understanding of the experiences of health and illness.

Institutions and therapies for depression offer an intimacy and a physical connection that might be exploited for its narrative potential. For example, even as Slater proclaims that "[p]sychopharmacology is the one branch of medicine where there is no need for intimacy," she describes the "Prozac Doctor" as "handsome in ways you don't expect your medicine man to be."[26] She details her relationship with Prozac in frankly sexual terms, summarizing her eventual relationship to the drug by writing: "Prozac is not my lover any longer but over the very long haul has become a close friend, a slightly anemic, well-meaning buddy whose presence can considerably ease pain but cannot erase it."[27]

The physical intimacy between drug and body parallels the psychic intimacy between illness and identity. Metaphors for depression run the risk of ultimately collapsing into themselves, reinforcing illness identities that fundamentally define individuals. Nevertheless, they may also provide the means by which individuals can write their own stories of health and illness, as Slater does. Her memoir could be described as a dialogical engagement with multiple discourses of health and illness, but her primary attention, indicated even by her title, is with the pharmaceutical treatment of her *self*. Slater's diary is a chronicle of and to herself (and her readers), but it is a chronicle that understands herself through the lens of Prozac. The drug's prominence in the story of her life shows it to be intimately connected to her sense of self, but it also brings with it mechanical metaphors and explanations for her illness. The scud missile is, after all, a technological advance over earlier weaponry; Prozac similarly replaces earlier pharmaceutical therapies. Nevertheless, Prozac and its mode of action rely on the cause-and-effect logic of neurotransmitter deficit and correction, both of which are isolated and isolating processes. While Slater's narrative draws on multiple discourses of health and illness, much of the discourse of depression remains focused on simplistic mechanical models.

Objectifying the Self

Mechanical models for depression promise to separate subjective emotions from objective science and chemistry. They bracket off most of the affective realities of the illness in favor of attending to the underlying causes that ostensibly precipitate those feelings. In the process, they dismiss the importance of depression's effects and focus on internal, causal factors; they alienate individuals from their own experiences. These constructions obviously favor particular solutions and responses to depression, as Joshua Wulf Shenk explains: "Phrases like 'running out of gas,' 'neurotransmitter deficits,' 'biochemical malfunctions,' and 'biological brain disease' are terribly common, and are favored by well-intentioned activists who seek parity between emotional and somatic illnesses. Pharmaceutical companies also like machine imagery, since they manufacture the oils, coolants, and fuels that are supposed to make us run without knocks or stalls."[28] Two communities are helped by the mechanical metaphors for depression: activists seeking parity between physical and mental illnesses and pharmaceutical companies who offer "repairs" via their medications. The issue of parity is a complicated one, as the discussion in chapter 3 suggested, and to base claims for it solely on a chemical etiology brushes aside a number of other possible arguments rooted in disability and social functioning. Curiously, the "serotonin hypothesis"—the impetus for many mechanical metaphors—has been discredited and largely rejected by scientists, who understand depression, to the extent that they do, as a product of far more complicated and interrelated mechanisms.[29] Nevertheless, the simplified hypothesis continues to generate mechanical metaphors and public understandings of depression as a matter of a few unbalanced chemicals that may be regulated via pharmaceutical intervention. Such constructions isolate depression within individuals' neurochemical systems, and they additionally shape the available illness identities through the specific forms they inhabit.

Mechanical metaphors might make use of a variety of activities—from the automotive examples in Shenk's description, to the intricacies of computer chip construction—but within the discourse of depression, they most often reside in domestic spaces. In Sara Rosenthal's self-help book *Women and Depression*, the serotonin hypothesis receives explanation by comparison to an inadequate laundry facility. She writes: "A simple analogy is to imagine that this system of brain chemistry exchange is like a washing machine. Serotonin is the 'water' that flows in at certain times and is flushed out. Normally, enough water flows in and out, and the machine functions properly. But, depression is akin to low water pressure. It would be like setting your washing machine on high only to find that the water level doesn't go beyond low."[30] Here, the discussion of the brain as a washing machine has several important implications. If we trace the metaphoric domains suggested by this analogy, the mind becomes not simply an appliance, but a particularly gendered one. Depression is, here, the fault of "low water pressure" and comes as a surprise to the operator who sets "the machine on high only to find that the water level doesn't go beyond low." Here the embedded difficulties—a mechanical problem of "low water pressure" and a cognitive problem of not *knowing* that one's machine cannot fill properly—work to encourage practices of self-doctoring first as matters of straightforward material repairs, and then as matters of faulty self-comprehension.

The analogy implies that a "work around" might be possible if one had advance knowledge of the water pressure situation, for example, by attempting smaller loads of laundry until the mechanic has visited. Reading the analogy in this way demonstrates its power to shape not only the concept of depression as an imbalance of neurochemicals but also to encourage self-knowledge and anticipation of potential problems. The laundry explanation assumes that serotonin levels—like the water in the machine—are regulated on demand, according to predictable cycles rather than being variable and unique to each individual brain. As a consequence, more serotonin (water pressure) is assumed to be the singular solution, even though current scientific knowledge suggests a more complicated correlation. Further, the domestic space in which this analogy operates contributes to the gendering and the privatizing of the illness. Laundry is a task performed at home (stereotypically by women) or in a laundromat, a designated public space that sanctions this private activity. Popular idioms such as an injunction against "airing one's dirty laundry in public" imply that public discussion of, in this case, one's depression might be shameful, particularly when the brain-as-washing-machine fails to operate efficiently. Depression, like laundry, should—in the terms of this analogy—be taken care of privately. Rosenthal's explanation attempts to familiarize her female audience with depression, but it also orients readers toward their own internal functioning and toward the gendered and moral judgments made about their external performances.

Another mechanical metaphor describes the action of the newer pharmaceuticals as if they were "keys" fitting into "locks" on specific receptors in the brain. Thompson describes the action of fluxoetine (Prozac) in just this way: "There, like a key fitting into a lock, the fluxoetine molecules slid into a spot on the neuron normally reserved for serotonin. That blocked serotonin molecules from being reabsorbed, increasing the number available in the synapse. . . . [T]his was a pill that jangled my brain juices."[31] In this construction, the drug fits neatly into the lock on the receptor, though it performs a duty dissimilar from a normal key. Whereas a key would be expected to *open* a door, in this case it keeps the serotonin from slipping back through the keyhole. The "neat" fit between pharmaceutical and receptor implies a custom solution, and the whole description promises personal security as well as mechanical functionality. In a *Newsweek* article, another analogy situates a treatment based on Omega-3 fatty acids within the home. "'Think of the receptor as a doorbell on a house,' says Dr. Lauren Marengell of Baylor College of Medicine. 'Omega-3s provide the lubrication that frees up a stuck doorbell and allows it to respond to a messenger's touch.'"[32] Here, the active agent lubricates, rather than blocks, activity in the brain, but it nevertheless performs a household (as opposed to public or corporate) repair. More significantly, this explanation renders human agency entirely secondary to the mechanical system: the messenger is useless until the mechanics are resolved. In this example, Omega-3 fatty acids promise to restore responsiveness to social communication. In the images of locks and doorbells, drug action is private and interior; in both images, the solution is an invasion of the self that promises to free one's responses to outsiders. The mechanisms of unlocking and unblocking suggest a return to social interactions via supplementation: both "jangled . . . brain juices" and a functioning doorbell invite a party into the private space of the individual. Beyond their implied messages about the illness, such metaphors describe the healthy ideal: an individual who is hospitable, receptive, and whose social functioning is smooth and effortless. To display health, then, individuals must attend to their social behaviors; to be ill is to be excluded from society.

Chemical explanations for depression have all of the modern trappings of scientific objectivity and have repressed the more naturalistic notions of balance common to humoral or homeopathic paradigms. Rather than a whole-body approach to illness, the chemical metaphor for depression is focused singularly on neurotransmitters. The pharmaceuticals developed to correct the assumed imbalances are seen as acting solely on the receptor sites of the nerve cells in the brain. Fixing the machine of the brain—even through chemical bombardment—becomes the primary object, leaving out discussions of rebuilding or fortifying the society that fostered the malfunction in the first place. Slater's military attack from afar requires precise geographies of the intended target, and these rhetorical constructions internalize the practice of mapping. The individual body becomes a target to be located and ameliorated. The 2001 Zoloft advertisement—with its dramatization of the malfunction pictured as an unpopulated gap between neurons—locates depression at the most microscopic level. Recent advertisements and a Web site for Cymbalta offer an education in the "Science of Depression," which includes a linear representation of two neurotransmitter systems—both serotonin and norepinephrine "pathways" are affected by the drug—within the body. On the Cymbalta Web site, an abstract and transparent torso contains blue and green chemical arteries that arch up the spine and curl into the brain. In this image, depression lurks along the linear pathways that connect brain to body, and it can be avoided by optimizing the neurological traffic.

Such mapping not only reduces depression to a chemical or mechanical problem, it also encourages suspicion of the body, which may harbor the illness and define the self as fundamentally ill. Drawing maps of and on the body reinforces connections between metaphoric constructions of depression as an enemy territory to be occupied and overwhelmed and the physical self, which becomes the front line of the battle. Because these pharmaceuticals promise (in their promotional advertising) to return individuals to themselves, these maps begin to shape not only what counts as illness, but also what should be expected of health. According to John Shilb, the extensive popular use of and talk about such medications provoke even nondepressed individuals to question the relationship between the self and brain chemistry.[33] If, in the words of one advertising campaign, a child can "get her mommy back" through the ingestion of Effexor, then perhaps all fundamental identities are vulnerable to or could benefit from chemical manipulations.

The twin practices of the *use* of pharmaceuticals and of the *discussion* surrounding them have not only characterized the recent history of depression, but they have shaped notions of selfhood as well. The self now inhabits a neurochemical territory and can be enhanced through additions to and subtractions from that chemical landscape. Indeed, the self can be comprehended in retrospect once a particular compound has achieved a desired effect. Such late twentieth-century practices of personal geography operate in reverse, from destination (cure) to route (illness), a process that Jennifer Radden calls "drug cartography."[34] When a particular compound labeled an *antidepressant* relieves symptoms, the illness is discovered to have been *depression*.

This process—whereby, for example, SSRIs have been found to be effective in a variety of illnesses from obsessive-compulsive disorder to depression to anxiety disorders—suggests relationships among entities that respond to the same interventions. The science begins to operate in response to drug reactions rather than first seeking plausible etiologies and then developing pharmaceutical interventions. In the era of the human genome project, practices of mapping and description have taken on paramount significance, perhaps at the expense of practices of healing and understanding.

Within my corpus, several reports concern viral, genetic, and biological hypotheses for the causes of depression. In these reports, as in the correlations between heart disease and depression, the exact relationship between physical system, mechanism of action, and illness is murky at best. Yet the speculation continues from remedy (for example, Omega-3 fatty acids) to cause (poorly developed brain tissue as precipitator of depression and heart disease), and the resulting conceptual frames develop accordingly. Such maps give the illusion of precision but fail to examine multiple interacting factors and realities. The utility of drug cartographies, however, has not been universally accepted. The skeptical view, as it is expressed by sociologist David Karp, argues that the fact that "people sometimes feel better after taking antidepressant medications is hardly definitive evidence that depression is caused by an underlying physical pathology. Such logic would require us to say that the individual who feels better after a glass or two of wine with dinner was de facto suffering from some biological impairment corrected by alcohol."[35] Nevertheless, conceptualizations of depression based in brain chemistry and assumed transmitter imbalances are both compelling and prevalent within the discourse of depression.

In my interview with the mental health professionals, Laurie describes with considerable appreciation and even envy an "elegant and easy" study of "just basal levels of serotonin in the brain." The study, she reports, finds that "men have more serotonin in the brain than women . . . and, so if there's going to be a deficit of serotonin at some point, if you already start low, you're going to be in more trouble." As she describes this study, Laurie uses an unusual number of adjectives to express her enthusiasm for the work, calling the study "elegant," "elegant and easy," and "this wonderful study." These adjectives evidence her desire for a simple, straightforward solution to the problem of depression, and her faith in the neurochemical model for depression. Even though her comments elsewhere indicate a skeptical orientation toward pharmaceutical intervention, Laurie's attitude here suggests a strong affiliation with mechanical models for depression.

For individuals who are experiencing some of the symptoms of depression, one very serious consequence of the mechanical models for depression is a faith in the ability of medicine to accurately judge and repair their damaged systems. Among one group of such women with whom I talked, the phrase "chemical imbalance" was used several times. After the women used this phrase, I asked the group how they would know if they had a chemical imbalance. Mei responded: "I don't know how to diagnose it [laughs], so . . . I don't know. I mean, aren't there some tests they could do?" This response is important for several reasons. First, Mei abdicates all authority over the mechanics of her brain. She assumes that if a chemical imbalance exists, then there are both tests to locate it and medications to correct it. Understanding the implications of "imbalance"—that a proper and discernible "balance" exists and can be accurately deciphered by experts—Mei has taken on the subjectivity available to her as a patient within the discourse of depression. In addition, her laughter indicates a sense of nervousness about being asked what she perceives to be a question requiring medical expertise. She and the others in the group claim "not to be shrinks," and, to this extent, the illness remains the province of experts assumed to have knowledge of the mechanics of the brain. Mei's desire for "tests" to determine the presence or absence of the correct balance of brain chemicals suggests that she sees science mapping both the illness and her own biochemistry. She assumes standards against which her own individual results might be read; she hopes for an easy legend for interpreting those results.

Women like Mei appear comfortable with the chemical and mechanical metaphors for depression. They are not, however, entirely ready to submit themselves to pharmaceutical treatment. Instead, they adopt other portions of the illness identity that require self-help and individual healing. Stephanie, for example, resists her mother's suggestion of using what Stephanie calls a "grow light" to combat symptoms of seasonal affective disorder. Stephanie says: "I don't think I'm desperate enough to go that route, 'cause I still think I can fix myself. I seem to think it's a character flaw rather than a clinical thing." About twenty minutes later, Stephanie repeats this sentiment, saying, "Well, I honestly do think I have a chemical imbalance sometimes, but I, like I say, I think I should be able to deal with it myself." In this second utterance, Stephanie accepts a definition of herself based in brain chemistry, but rejects the consequent action (taking medication, using a light box) in favor of other forms of self-doctoring available to her. In another group of women, the discussion of "chemical" etiologies of depression is dismissed as too simple. Paige, a senior humanities major, speaks scornfully of the drug advertisements that seem to offer easy solutions. When Claire, a master's of arts student, challenges Paige by asking, "What if it's [i.e., depression is] chemical?" Paige responds:

PAIGE: It *is* chemical. I mean, like, I don't know biology enough to know . . . the neurological processes. . . . [But] it's clear that there's something in my mind, a chemical process in the mind that has something to do with the way I feel, because that's what . . . the chemical equivalent of emotions is. . . . If you can convince yourself to be happy there's a chemical process that goes with that, and if you can convince yourself to change . . . the ways you think or the things that you do . . . that's also a chemical process. So, it's a chemical solution, the same as taking a pill.

For both Paige and for Stephanie, the underlying relevance of a "chemical theory" of depression is valid enough, but there is *more* than a simple chemical solution. Both women seem to believe that there is other work to be done, and that the illness cannot fully be contained by a mechanical understanding. Depression is still, as Stephanie claims, viewed as a "character flaw"—as something innate, shameful, and ultimately one's individual burden to bear—rather than a sterile "clinical thing." The self remains complicit even when models that seem to address a more physical body are accepted. The discourse of depression fosters a variety of foundational metaphors and understandings of the illness. Just as definitional practices reveal a strategic imprecision that compels self-doctoring, metaphoric and figurative explanations encourage the development of versions of the self that comply with expectations for social interaction. When the self cannot integrate, the illness must be eradicated by the individual in isolation.

Indistinct boundaries between "chemical" and "emotional" depressions are maintained within the discourse as added impetus for practices of self-doctoring. While mechanical models might seem to absolve individuals of responsibility, other possibilities—that the self is to blame for its own troubles—seem to trap women in particular. Danquah describes the conundrum:

Often I am asked whether the depressions I have are emotional or bio-chemical. Having posed that question to myself a million times before, I am well aware of its implications, that an emotional depression is less profound, more topical because it is issue-related, and has very little to do with one's brain chemistry. As all our emotions and moods are bio-chemically induced, regardless of whether the prompts are internal or external, this supposition is false. All clinical depressions are a mixture of the emotional and the biochemical; the illness exists somewhere in that ghost space between consciousness and chemistry.[36]

Here, she writes of a "ghost space" that includes both "consciousness and chemistry," drawing the chemical analogy into the amorphous realm of the self. The question of responsibility becomes confused with such "mixtures" of self and chemistry, and therefore the self becomes a site of constant surveillance and monitoring. Danquah has questioned herself "a million times" about her illness, evidence of her extensive self-monitoring and anxiety.

The results of such self-scrutiny seem to be practices of intense self-doctoring. For example, after she begins taking Prozac, Slater describes her "cure" as a process of being tuned as if she were a musical instrument. She writes: "It was as though I'd been visited by a blind piano tuner who had crept into my apartment at night, who had tweaked the ivory bones of my body, the taut strings in my skull, and now, when I pressed on myself, the same notes but with a mellower, fuller sound sprang out."[37] Coming out of depression requires relearning oneself. For Slater and for Danquah, this modification of the *self* occurs through pharmaceutical intervention, but the illness remains intimately attached to their personal identities. Mechanical metaphors of washing machines and doorbells dissolve into speculations about the self and its personal responsibility for social functioning; military metaphors invoke pharmaceutical or bureaucratic campaigns against individuals; chemistry appears to offer the simple explanation, but it fails to account for the whole experience of depression, leaving individuals to blame themselves for incomplete solutions. In effect, mechanical metaphors offer obviously simplistic solutions that target desires for social reconnection while shifting responsibility onto the individual for achieving those ends.

Internalizing Geographies

As the notion of a drug cartography suggests, spatial metaphors and those implying travel and exploration are highly productive within the discourse of depression. The conceptual metaphor LIFE IS A JOURNEY can indeed be seen to structure many responses to depression, including viewing the illness as a diversion or detour along life's pathway. The illness itself is often represented as a territory into which one is led by a variety of paths and out of which pharmaceutical routes are sometimes taken.[38] Recalling Susan Sontag's kingdoms of the healthy and the ill, such metaphors for depression are not unique among figurative responses to illness.[39] But, within these metaphors of place and space, both the depressed individual and the illness are subject to exploration. Whether neurochemical pathways are implicated in depression or the illness leads one into new terrain, the efforts of mapping attend both to the self and to the illness. As much as the illness occupies a space—the topographical and sociological area detailed in, for example, Solomon's subtitle to *The Noonday Demon: An Atlas of Depression*—that space quickly moves from exterior landscapes to the interior spaces of buildings and, eventually, the self. "Depression," Manning writes, "carries no papers. It enters your country unannounced and uninvited. Its origins are unknown, but its destination always dead-ends in you."[40] Here *you* are both the wide territory, invaded by depression as an unannounced visitor, and also the destination, the final stop for illness. In other versions, depression remaps the world from within an individual. Rather than dead-ending in a singular self, depression in Jeffrey Smith's description transports the self into a new world. He writes: "All we can say with any certainty is that no matter its divergent origins and pathways, the eventual expression of melancholia results from biochemical changes in the brain. . . . Those hard-worn pathways will deliver you onto one broad thoroughfare, the encompassing experience we call clinical depression. On the brain there is some new map. . . . It remakes the world."[41] Smith's new world is not a physically unique place; it is a new topography of the brain. The biochemical pathways that "deliver you onto" depression's "broad thoroughfare" are interior routes traveled in isolation and largely without consciousness. Within the discourse of depression, the self is something to be mapped, studied, and traversed. These geographies, as Smith's description demonstrates, move back and forth across the borders between internal *self* and external *world*, but they tend to come to rest in the singular and solitary individual.

When depression is located outside of the self, it becomes a new territory to be navigated, primarily without a guide. How one arrives in this new and dangerous location is a matter of traveling any of a variety of paths, some of which are thoroughfares—"victimization is a sure path to depression"[42]—and others are complex networks that connect to other afflictions of the body, for example, the "number of possible pathways . . . [and] multiple channels by which depression and heart disease are linked."[43] Such movement into depression encourages spatial understandings of the illness, but not only are the routes unmarked, the destination itself resists mapping. Manning describes her hospitalization for depression as a loss of citizenship in her old life. She writes: "Being hospitalized on a psychiatric unit was, for me, like crossing over into a different state. I've lost citizenship in the old place, but I haven't totally settled into the new one either. . . . To know the force of the avalanche and my powerlessness over it is to feel myself in brand-new territory."[44] Her powerlessness over herself transports her irrevocably beyond the familiar and comfortable geographies of health. Her new territory appears uncharted, however, and she, like Slater, must create her own map even as she feels powerless to do so.

Recovery, as Manning's and Slater's memoirs detail, is another pathway within the territory of depression, but it is a route that also appears without landmarks or signposts. In one NIMH brochure directed toward men, retired U.S. Air Force sergeant Patrick McCathern speaks of the slow journey toward health as one that becomes visible only in hindsight. The brochure quotes him directly: "Pretty soon you start having good thoughts about yourself and that you're not worthless and you kind of turn your head over your shoulder and look back at that, that rutted, muddy, dirt road that you just traveled and now you're on some smooth asphalt and go, 'Wow, what a trip. Still got a ways to go, but I wouldn't want to go down that road again.'"[45] The experience of depression—the road he would not care to travel again—appears uncivilized (a rutted dirt road), and a return to health is characterized by the smooth asphalt of modern society. Such images isolate the illness beyond the reach of social aid; the infrastructure is inadequate to support relief work. The journey toward health is elsewhere characterized as a process of maturation: small steps lead eventually to a return of adult functioning. For example: "Micro-steps are the beginning of a journey. Like a toddler, you have to crawl before you can walk. And you have to get used to falling down and picking yourself up again. Eventually you will be able to take charge of your life again."[46] These examples posit depression as an unknown and isolated territory, requiring difficult and solitary travel (back) toward social functioning. Health, by comparison, once it is achieved is imagined as a straightforward experience, a familiar path. After the pain of illness and the arduous journey of healing, health is simply described as being "on track."[47]

Within the complex geography of depression, however, we might begin to locate a rhetorical care of the self that acknowledges the diverse territories of health *and* illness. Rather than imagining healing as a rebirth or a return to civilization, such self-care might work to map the overlapping territories of health and illness, perhaps discovering that they are not nearly as isolated or independent as we might wish to think. In my interviews with women experiencing symptoms of depression, each woman expresses some dissatisfaction with her life. In many cases, this dissatisfaction takes the metaphorical shape of standing at a crossroad, wondering which path to choose: they discuss the notion of "lacking a direction in your life." For example, Jennifer mentions wanting to seek out a mental health professional to gain a new perspective. She concludes that she might be "reaching to the point" where she is willing to consult an "expert." She talks explicitly about the numerous paths that she feels she is choosing among: "Maybe I have the solutions and I've thought about them, but I haven't—I just don't actively do them, because I just want somebody else to tell me that it's okay, . . . that this is, you know, what you should do. This is the path you should take. . . . I might have three different paths and I'm just not sure which one, you know." Jennifer characterizes herself as at a particular location ("the point") and as wanting someone to "guide me to do the right thing to get me out of it." In this statement, she opens herself to the potential of assistance, though she couches her desire for guidance with a deferential attitude toward "a professional." Nevertheless, she seems ready to engage with a therapeutic intervention that might explore multiple paths and directions—this seems a promising sign of potential self-care.

Beyond this form of self-location, the women in my interviews refer to taking medications for depression as "going down that route." In one interview, Claire relates a friend's experiences on Prozac, which make her "fearful of taking Prozac and I was like, 'there's got to be another way besides drugs.'" Here, she talks about wanting an alternative to drug therapy, another "way" to proceed. Similarly, Jennifer talks about the medications, saying, "They're a lot better now than they once were, but I didn't really want to go that route just yet." In both cases, the women do not see the "route" of drug therapy as a currently viable option, but both women see it as a potential direction. I read these references to routes and pathways as potentially hopeful—the women are visualizing options for themselves and their futures, and they seem to be balancing and exploring a number of possible responses to their experiences. These moments represent potential sites of intervention and pedagogy—the women are asking for multiple options, even though the discourse offers primarily pharmaceutical solutions. Perhaps Jennifer's desire to talk to a mental health professional might open a dialogue, potentially offering her discursive tools with which to navigate her future.

THE CARTOGRAPHY of depression narrows from natural territories to architectural layouts, mirroring a similar constriction from world travels to internal, biochemical pathways. For example, the mechanical analogy of the doorbell works only in the frame of a house and, surprisingly, visitors. In addition, several descriptions of depression use the metaphoric construction of buildings and rooms. A *Newsweek* story detailing the suicide of Native American author Michael Dorris quotes his wife, Louise Erdrich, describing her husband's "public cheerfulness '[as] only the third floor of a building with a very deep basement.'"[48] In this description, depression occupies the "very deep basement" of Dorris's emotional range, and from these depths, the logic of his suicide emerges. Here, depression is hidden, underground, and it is also at the very foundation of his personality. Similarly, for Styron, depression had been "hidden away for so long somewhere in the dungeons of my spirit."[49] These "dungeons" and "basements" clearly take their force from the orientational metaphor DOWN IS BAD, but they also call to mind physical, human, and private structures.

For Tipper Gore, wife of former-presidential candidate Al Gore, a revelation that she had suffered from depression led to a number of additional questions from the media. One *Newsweek* article, titled "Tipper Gore Keeps Cautious Watch at Door She Opened," paints her as profoundly secretive about her illness.[50] The opened "door" exists between Gore's public and private lives. She is characterized as "cautious" but also as having invited the attention (having opened the door herself). Similarly, a review of Andrew Solomon's *Noonday Demon* offers the following "highlight" summary: "A writer's journey into the dark corners of despair we call depression illuminates more than his condition."[51] The process of writing is here a journey into "dark corners"—depression is a building—but it is also an illumination of *more* than the "condition" itself. In descriptions of Gore and of Solomon's book, a sense of voyeurism constructs the available subjectivities for sufferers of the illness: they become territories to be explored and invaded by drugs, by others' attention, and by their own revelations.

Personal and constructed spaces—corners, basements, dungeons—cast depression as a private and human (as opposed to natural) condition. Despite various evolutionary models that seem to account for the presence of depression within the gene pool, there is still a sense of personal responsibility when one suffers from the illness. Some of this responsibility derives from the sheer number of denials deemed necessary in texts that confess or describe depression: the "not-statements" in chapter 3, as well as outright assertions of memoirists that they have struggled long and hard against the illness. But the conceptual metaphor of personal spaces helps reinforce the individual isolation and responsibility that accrues to depression. In Thompson's memoir, she describes mental illness as "a kind of exile into a foreign territory of the mind, although this foreign territory is right next door. It is a room—imagine it as plain white, featureless, empty—which most people may not enter, and from which others may never leave."[52] The blankness and the proximity of the territory "right next door" help to contain depression, when it can no longer be exiled, and both features locate depression in the *mind* rather than in the world.

For Solomon, depression reflects the decay of one's structural integrity; he writes:

> You go along the gradual path or the sudden trigger of emotion and then you get to a place that is genuinely different. It takes time for a rusting iron-framed building to collapse, but the rust is ceaselessly powdering the solid, thinning it, eviscerating it. The collapse, no matter how abrupt it may feel, is the cumulative consequence of decay. It is nonetheless a highly dramatic and visibly different event. It is a long time from the first rain to the point when rust has eaten through an iron girder. Sometimes the rusting is at such key points that the collapse seems total, but more often it is partial: this section collapses, knocks that section, shifts the balances in a dramatic way.[53]

The cause-and-effect language of Solomon's description takes the form of ecology—rain falling on a building—but the damage is to human and social constructions. The shifts in balance Solomon reports are shifts that occur because underlying structures have been weakened by "the cumulative consequence of decay." Decay of one's inner supports—the girders of one's self— makes one vulnerable to the illness. Manning describes the fear of depression rendering her "terrified that I will be drawn like a magnet back down those dark stairs and long halls to that awful time and place and self."[54] This fear—lurking at the edges of all depression memoirs—makes explicit the connection between the "dark stairs and long halls" and the "awful time and place and *self*" that depression entails. This, then, is a primary consequence of the discourse of depression—to create an anxiety about the self that requires constant observation and maintenance.

Spatial metaphors for depression take their logic from a notion of life as a journey through sometimes difficult terrain. Yet the forms of these metaphors work to contain the illness in foreign, isolated, or uncivilized territories. Failing that, additional metaphors locate depression in the domestic architecture of the self, thereby placing the burden of egress back on the individual. Figurative constructions imagine they can monitor the routes and pathways into and out of depression and thereby distance health from illness. In hindsight, however, the two territories clearly adjoin (if not overlap), and an attention to these communicating passages might encourage a more complex array of responses to depression. The reduction of territories to architecture, particularly when individuals themselves are rendered as buildings, promotes practices of self-doctoring—primarily suspicion of the self and its resulting vigilant monitoring—that might be transformed into tactics of self-care by illuminating the "dark corners" of the self and encouraging a more complete and flexible cartography that would locate *both* health and illness among multiple discourses rather than simply within the discourse of biological psychiatry.

Metaphoric Transmission

In an article discussing Tipper Gore's depression, the author reports that Gore "would not say precisely when depression struck. She would not say how long ago it lifted, or all the symptoms she exhibited, or what medication she took."[55] Framed as a litany of withheld information, this text highlights the extent to which *communication* about depression has become expected from those who suffer from it. Here, Gore herself becomes almost a museum, albeit one closed to the public, of her illness: her current behavior blocks the *exhibition* of her past symptoms, course of illness, and pharmaceutical therapies. Nevertheless, the text assumes these features to be part of the public presentation of her depression. In other words, despite Gore's refusal to provide details, her illness is still sketched for public review. Communication serves as both a literal and a figurative force within the discourse of depression, perhaps because the passing and receiving messages—both literal communication between individuals, and metaphorical chemical processes in the brain—defines human interaction.

Indeed, the word *transmit* originates as a verb describing the mechanical action of transporting something across space or time, but in the seventeenth century, it was figuratively applied in the sense of *communicating* something rather than physically transferring it. These two meanings are sufficiently common to support the use of both—the physical transportation of serotonin from one nerve cell to another, and the literate communication of symptoms within a medical consultation—in referring to depression. The 1949 Shannon and Weaver "mathematical model of communication" emphasizes the movement of a "message" between a "transmitter" and a "receiver."[56] Similarly, representations of neurons, such as the one found in a Life Balance publication titled *Depression*, label one neuron "transmitting" and the other "receiving."[57] Thus, a conflation between *communicating* and *transporting* appears a natural extension of the overlapping definitions. According to one *Newsweek* article, "Normal brain function involves the passage of *chemical messengers* between cells."[58] Similarly, regions of the brain are said to communicate with one another through such signals: "The right prefrontal cortex, for example, *communicates* with certain types of immune cells, and stress appears to alter the functioning of *a chemical messenger*, dopamine, in the region."[59] These neurotransmitters are personified as "mood-boosting messengers"[60] who can "touch" or activate a doorbell and set in motion the consequent interactions. Metaphoric descriptions suggest that depression is a matter of being incommunicative: a failure to make neurochemical connections mirrors a failure to perform socially.

In addition to the relay of messages, the notion of *communication* draws with it the possible taint of *contagion*. One article asserts that "like the flu, depression is a highly contagious disorder that can be transmitted socially, jumping from one family member to others. And just as individuals can be depressed, so can whole families, often without their awareness."[61] The insidious nature of an illness that individuals or family can have "without their awareness" adds a need for vigilance and self-monitoring. These suspicions are fostered within my corpus by statements such as "sometimes anxiety is dispositional, and sometimes it's transmitted to children by parental over-concern."[62] Imprecise qualifiers such as *sometimes* and the modal *can*, which carries less certainty than the future-tense marker *will*, postulate problems that must be guarded against, even if they are not assured of happening. Such discursively structured anxieties encourage practices of self-doctoring by suggesting that sufferers are responsible for safeguarding their families through a careful monitoring of themselves.

While clear communication is denied to sufferers of depression, and, indeed, the dangers of communicating anxiety and depression to one's family are restated, the illness and particularly its pharmaceutical treatments are sometimes couched in linguistic metaphors. Manning describes her depression as a loss of language: "I have lost [my friends'] language, their facility with words that convey feelings."[63] For Solomon, depression acts as a ventriloquist when a friend stops him by saying, "That's the depression talking. It's talking through you."[64] Manning and Solomon have been silenced by illness; the medications they ingest, however, seem to have gained voice, or at least the ability to convey meaning. Solomon writes: "Every morning and every night, I look at the pills in my hand: white, pink, red, turquoise. Sometimes they seem like writing in my hand, hieroglyphics saying that the future may be all right and that I owe it to myself to live on and see."[65] Though the pills appear to be in an unknown and ancient language, they nevertheless convey hope, sanity, and a sense of future, which Solomon himself has lost. Similarly, for Slater, her first prescription for Prozac appears to her to be undecipherable, yet it conveys the sense of "a plea" or prayer for her own future. The Prozac Doctor, she writes, "handed me the piece of paper. I folded it into tiny squares and shoved it in my knapsack. Later on, when I unfolded it, I felt like I was unwrapping a tiny present, or a plea, something slipped inside the Wailing Wall, written in a language I could little understand."[66] In these ways, communication comes to animate the illness and its cures, while it remains elusive for individuals themselves.

Metaphors of communication—between pharmaceuticals and patients, along chemical pathways in the brain, between individuals suffering from depression and their doctors, friends, and acquaintances—serve to repopulate the landscape of depression, but they do so in highly restricted forms. "Talk to your doctor" is a phrase that inevitably references chemical solutions to depression. Nevertheless, the metaphors—not just of communication, but also of animals, mechanics, and spaces—for depression provide a rich space for engaging the illness from within the discourse itself. As Jennifer's comments suggest, the usefulness of a *journey* metaphor might lie in its ability to encourage an individual to consider multiple options. The animal familiars that haunt depression might serve as models for a social recognition of the illness—the *family* dog, rather than *my* dog—that could encourage broader practices of self-care. Even the mechanical constructions have important social potential to promote parity between physical and mental illnesses. Yet none of these figures of depression can be deployed tactically unless they are understood as part of a broad and multivocal discursive framework.

The power of metaphor lies in its ability to evoke narrative: mechanical models are hardly coercive until one comprehends the whole *story* of the broken washing machine, the likely causes of its dysfunction, and its necessary repairs. Such elaborated stories of depression—those told in memoirs and the brief exemplary narratives within public discourse—offer opportunities to explore the structuration of the illness. Whereas metaphors seem to isolate individuals and thereby encourage their deployment of self-doctoring practices, narratives offer images of acceptable identities—often explicitly gendered identities—that serve as models toward which individuals are encouraged to perform. Together, metaphors and narratives of depression give form to the illness and the subjectivities available in relation to it. A rhetorical care of the self, therefore, must adopt critical reading strategies that open opportunities for the tactical use of the images and the stories those images might evoke within the discourse.

5

Telling Stories of Depression

Models for the Gendered Self

Metaphors for depression focus attention relentlessly inward: broad geographies narrow to personal drug cartographies, mythic beasts rarely replace familiars and domestic companions, mechanical descriptions illuminate the microscopic spaces between neurons. The larger stories in which these figurative constructions are embedded work in similar ways to direct individual attention toward the self, particularly toward the gendered self. Within stories of depression, specifically gendered forms of self-doctoring are modeled and prescribed to readers. Built on the foundations of imprecise definitional practices, isolating metaphors, and the science of biological psychiatry, stock characters in these stories encourage self-fashioning within restricted health and illness identities and sanction traditional modes of social interaction. Isolated individuals—encouraged to monitor their practices of the self—are, within stories, invited back into social scenes, but those scenes offer only traditional gender roles and responsibilities. The discourse of depression both reflects and shapes larger cultural discourses about gender: it draws on familiar archetypes (the overworked male executive, the unhappy housewife), but it also recirculates those archetypes and the story lines that accompany them. Such discursive recirculation helps shape depression as a "woman's illness," and it suggests the need for responsive self-doctoring practices from *both* men and women.

In 2005, the Zoloft creature, who sat alone in the darkness in the 2001 advertisement (figure 3), returns to print advertising within the frames of a simple graphic narrative. "This is Kathy's Story," proclaims the 2005 image, heralding a significant shift in perspective away from the lonely creature and toward the promise of social interaction (figure 8). Stories, after all, require both narrators and audiences. In the persona of "Kathy," the creature becomes an actor within a story rather than a static representation of the depressed self. This shift is evident in the sentence patterns of each advertisement: second-person assertions

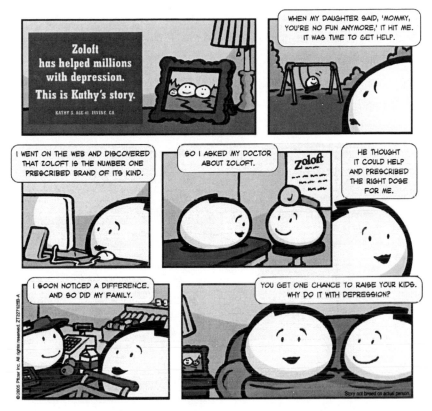

Kathy researched all the medications. She found out that ZOLOFT has helped millions with depression and anxiety. ZOLOFT is safe and effective. It has treated more people with more types of depression and anxiety than any brand of its kind. So she asked her doctor about ZOLOFT. ZOLOFT. #1 for millions of reasons.

Zoloft (sertraline HCl)
www.zoloft.com

FIGURE 8. Zoloft advertisement, 2005. (*Redbook*, February 2005)

characterize the earlier text ("You know when you're not feeling like yourself"); first-person reports of self-doctoring activities occur in the 2005 version ("I went on the Web and discovered . . ."). There is a variety of factors contributing to this shift from authoritative assertions toward personal narratives. In the years between 2001 and 2005, the science of biological psychiatry came under additional scrutiny and criticism, leading to more complex questions about the mechanisms of illness such as depression. Studies found an increase in suicidal behaviors in adolescents prescribed drugs such as Zoloft, and the FDA responded in 2004 by requiring a "black box" warning to accompany advertisements for those drugs.[1] In addition to these increased suspicions, however, the discourse itself seems to have absorbed the chemical imbalance model for depression to such an extent that the model itself was no longer novel enough to merit explanation in advertising. Rhetorical energy began to focus more explicitly on treatment *outcomes*—the return to selfhood promised all along by the pharmaceutical companies—rather than the chemical processes that were intended to produce them.

In addition to returning selfhood to depressed individuals, these advertisements seem to promise a rearticulation of the healthy self, particularly the gendered self. The story within the 2005 Zoloft advertisement transforms "Kathy" into a perfect wife and mother via her activities of self-doctoring.[2] The end result of such self-doctoring takes center stage in relation to potential depression and also in relation to desired forms of health. Storytelling demonstrates *how* the drugs inspire in more socially embedded forms of self-monitoring: in Kathy's story, motherhood is being modeled as much as an illness is being treated. Each frame reiterates the power of depression to be a catalyst for self-doctoring in the late twentieth century. Kathy seeks help after her daughter, who is pictured happily swinging in the distant background of the first frame, tells her that she is "no fun anymore." Her daughter's judgment—another's report that might serve as diagnostic evidence within the context of the *DSM* definition—is the impetus for Kathy's self-doubt. Her self-diagnosis occurs in the next two frames, as she consults two expert systems: her computer (connected to online health information) and her physician. Both consultations require Kathy to assume the subjectivity of a depressed patient. Further, they are both straightforwardly medication-driven: on the Web, Kathy finds "that Zoloft is the number one prescribed brand of its kind" and in the doctor's office (where the physician sits smiling in front of a Zoloft poster), she asks about the medication specifically. The act of prescription—which traditionally represents the doctor's authority and power—is recounted in an unframed square of the graphic narrative; it is revealed by Kathy and *outside* of the doctor's office. In a move that mimics an actor's direct address to the audience, Kathy tells readers that "he [the doctor is stereotypically male] thought it [Zoloft] could help." Kathy has become the spokesperson for her own medical treatment; her doctor does not speak at all. In fact, his reported speech grants him only limited authority: he *thought* the drug *could* help. Both the indication of the physician's belief (instead of his certainty) and the possibility (but not necessity) implied by the modal *could* suggest that the diagnosis is not certain. It is for Kathy, however. She displays a single-minded focus on and confidence in the diagnosis and the treatment (via Zoloft) that results from her own self-doctoring.

Recovery, in Kathy's story, signals a return to social functioning, but within a gendered and domestic setting. Kathy displays explicit markers of gender—a fuller, lipsticked mouth—and narrates her experience only in relation to the gender-specific roles available. After taking Zoloft, Kathy and her family notice a difference (she is, presumably, fun again), which she reports while purchasing the family groceries. The final frame of the story shows Kathy and her husband seated on a couch. She is facing forward (addressing the reader with her gaze); he is looking at her and smiling, marking her recovery as a reentry into the family, much as her daughter's complaints marked her illness as a failure to perform as a mother. Kathy says: "You get one chance to raise your kids. Why do it with depression?" She has resumed her traditional family and gender roles with the help of Zoloft, and her family appears to be returned to "normal." But, the question she asks readers—Why raise children with depression?— echoes the accusation of Cymbalta's campaign (Who does depression hurt?) that suggests that women are harming their children by failing to seek treatment for depression. Appropriate motherhood, in the context of these advertisements, requires acts of self-doctoring. Such acts engage with the discourse of depression online, in the doctor's office, and in negotiation with one's friends and family. Simply being "no fun" is enough to suggest a need to modify one's gendered performances of the self; requesting medication returns the self to proper functioning.

The title frame of the Zoloft narrative declares: "This is Kathy's Story." It goes on to list demographic details: "Kathy S. Age: 41, Irvine, CA." In small letters in the bottom-right corner of the last frame of the narrative is the simple disclaimer: "Story not based on actual person." The initial assertion of personhood (Kathy owns her story) appears in white text on a medium-blue background; the disclaimer appears as its negative, in black text on the brown background of the couch. The story of this advertisement clearly seeks empathy and identification from readers, who may never notice the quasi-retraction at the end that declares the testimonial a fiction. The story persuades not through actual testimony, but through citation of key features of the discourse of depression. The veracity of Kathy's story is, in the final analysis, unimportant. She is most persuasive as a product of the discourse, performing all of the necessary acts of self-doctoring and achieving the desired result (pharmaceutical intervention and social reintegration). The advertisement constructs an ideal protagonist; it models a singular response to illness: a female patient who cannot perform her social duties comes to understand herself as depressed and takes medication to return herself to appropriate functioning. As this example demonstrates, stories of depression promise interpersonal connection— something too often lacking in the metaphoric constructions of the illness— and they offer strategies for self-doctoring that target gendered behaviors and social roles. Nevertheless, they might also be made to serve more tactical purposes if narrators and audiences can be encouraged to interrogate the scripts, rather than their own selves, more carefully. Such tactical uses of these stories are largely absent from my corpus of public texts, but the women whom I interviewed do offer small yet significant critiques of the storylines the discourse offers them. Nevertheless, their conversation reveals a strong bias toward gendered notions of emotionality and therefore susceptibility to depression. The stories of depression offer women and men models that encourage fine-tuned emotional self-monitoring in women and decisive action and a return to autonomy in men. In both cases, self-doctoring practices develop in the absence of more rhetorical approaches to self-care. By considering the stories and narrative impulses within the discourse of depression, perhaps such rhetorical critiques may produce more effective forms of self-care.

"A Steady Supply of Titles": The Narrative Impulse within the Discourse of Depression

The discursive production of selves depends on the dynamics of individual and collective disclosure: writers find readers who become writers of their own stories. Within book-length stories of depression, authors often explicitly describe such communicative exchanges. For example, in the author's note that prefaces *Darkness Visible*, William Styron traces the evolution of his text as a series of rhetorical occasions that respond both to his own need to retell his autobiography and to his audiences' continued interest in it. He explains that the text was first delivered as a lecture in Baltimore in May 1989, then revised rapidly for publication in *Vanity Fair* in December of that year. Neither version, however, provided Styron with enough space to include the narrative of a trip to Paris, which he felt had "special significance."[3] Wishing to revise his text and restore the Paris trip to "its place at the beginning," Styron pursued the publication of *Darkness Visible* in 1990. In his author's note, Styron portrays his own illness narrative as a work-in-progress, himself as consistently available for re-narration. He introduces the fact of a collective witnessing of his own illness across the series of texts he writes. Within the memoir itself, Styron reveals an additional antecedent text: his *New York Times* editorial that, in 1987, commented on the suicide of Primo Levi. Styron's editorial and each of the subsequent texts he writes can therefore be seen as conversational moves.

He responds to the texts that construct Levi's death as incomprehensible; he continues to respond to his own texts of self-revelation and readers' responses to them.

Beyond its personal significance to Styron, the conversation his texts enact gains momentum from the public reaction to each text. Styron describes the public response to his *New York Times* editorial as "spontaneous—and enormous."[4] Readers connect to his text and demonstrate their connection via additional texts (letters, stories) of their own. Styron concludes: "I had helped unlock a closet from which many souls were eager to come out and proclaim that they, too, had experienced the feelings I had described."[5] Styron's individual expression catalyzes a collective outpouring that, in turn, reinforces the rhetorical construction of the illness and the selves available in relation to it. In reading his text, Styron's audience feels authorized to share "the feelings [he] had described," and to express those feelings in additional stories. Styron characterizes these stories as *souls*, as individuals "eager to come out and proclaim" their illness identities. Indeed, Styron's book may be "defined by such moments of self-discovery and communal discovery," as critic Abigail Cheever concludes.[6] More than simply identifying the aesthetic structure of Styron's text, however, this formulation posits the close connections among the acts of writing, reading, and self-discovery.

Storytelling appears to be an integral part of the experience of depression, suggesting that depression is both an illness (the subject of one's writing) and an identity (the authority through which one writes). Styron's stated aim in *Darkness Visible* and elsewhere is to promote the understanding of depression as an illness, a disease that, he claims, robs individuals of their very selves. Yet even as he tells his story in order to reclaim his self, Styron is redefined around the illness; he emerges through the biochemistry of his illness, a figure articulated from within the discourse of depression. Elizabeth Wurtzel is perhaps the best known of the memoirists of the 1990s–2000s to exhibit a self defined by her own depression, but in many other cases, stories of depression offer new and gendered identities. These stories of selfhood replace fantasies of simple (chemical or surgical) cures; they are built on discursive foundations and reflect discursive pressures. Thus, they also represent potential sites for rhetorical intervention. Nevertheless, what is striking about the stories from this late twentieth-century period is their reliance on relatively simplistic identifications with rather than more critical revisions and elaborations of the depressed self.

Andrew Solomon's *Noonday Demon* remarks the magnitude of shared experience, but does so at the expense of providing a sense of individuality. Writing about how he compiled the stories that he includes in his text, Solomon remarks: "I met an enormous number of people in my ordinary life who volunteered, upon learning of my subject, their own copious histories, some of which were extremely fascinating and ultimately became source material. I published an article about depression in the *New Yorker* in 1998 and received over a thousand letters in the months immediately following publication."[7] The letters Solomon receives, much like the also "enormous" response to Styron's editorial on Levi's suicide, indicate the power of stories of depression to produce self-recognition and self-disclosure. That many of Solomon's subjects are drawn from his "ordinary life" and that these individuals "volunteered, upon learning of [his] subject, their own copious histories" testifies to the readiness of individuals to talk about the illness, even when given only the slight encouragement of a shared subject matter. Solomon receives the stories he is offered and translates them into "source material" out of which he constructs his own text. That text generalizes from the original stories in acts of repetition and translation that demonstrate the collective nature of individual expressions of the illness experience. To tell a personal story of depression is, it seems, to respond to and incorporate the stories of others, and thus, to author the self through a collective discourse.

Meri Nana-Ama Danquah traces the origins of her memoir, *Willow Weep for Me*, to a telephone conversation between herself and her *Washington Post* editor. Her retelling of these origins highlights the accommodations between author and audience within stories of depression. Initially considering the story of her illness not even worthy of publication, Danquah volunteers it simply as a response to her editor's question, "What've you been up to?" Launching into "an extremely long-winded anecdote," Danquah notes that the more her editor asks, the more she reveals about her struggle with depression. The conversation ultimately results in her public narrative; however, she must recast her story to accommodate and incorporate an audience already familiar with the discourse of depression. Having identified a publishable story for her from within her personal narrative, her editor offers Danquah writing advice:

> "There's a whole lot of stuff being written about depression these days. Have you read William Styron's book? If you were to write a piece, you'd have to make sure that you weren't repeating what's already been said, which will be pretty hard to do."
>
> "Yeah, right," I said sarcastically. "Like Styron and I would ever have the same angle on anything. We had the same illness; the similarities end there. The way I did depression was a-whole-nother bag of beans. I'm a single black mother about a half a paycheck away from the government cheese line."
>
> "There you have it," he said, as if he'd struck gold. "Make it about two thousand words, no more than twenty-five hundred. You can keep it personal, but you've gotta hook into what's going on out there. Remember to push the transcendence key. I've gotta run to a meeting. Call me if you get stuck. Bye."[8]

This exchange, which results not in a twenty-five-hundred word news feature but in a full-length depression memoir, displays some of the contradictions within the compulsive storytelling of depression. Cautioning her not to repeat "what's already been said," Danquah's editor nevertheless urges her to "hook into what's going on out there." She may "keep it personal" but must also "push the transcendence key." This advice emphasizes the need to speak to themes and topics familiar enough to the audience to indicate that this story participates in the genre already familiar to them. Further, the editor's comments reveal a lot about the public tastes for narratives: that they be generally positive (transcending the illness); that they be unique, but not so idiosyncratic as to ignore the common experience of depression; that they combine personal disclosure with collective witnessing, treading the fine line Solomon describes between the "literary pleasure of communication" and the "therapeutic release of self-expression."[9] In addition, the exchange foregrounds the collaborative nature of self-authoring. Danquah does not at first see her depression as newsworthy; her authorship is produced by the conversation in which her editor maps the discursive terrain which she will, in turn, have to navigate. The origins of Danquah's memoir reflect the complex interactions among previous texts, audience expectations, and authorial roles available within the discourse of depression; another place to trace these interactions is within responses to individuals' stories.

IN A REVIEW of Lewis Wolpert's *Malignant Sadness*, we learn that "most public libraries seem to need a steady supply of titles on depression, and this is recommended as the latest treatise on the subject."[10] Depression, in this analysis, appears an intrinsically rhetorical phenomenon, compelling new texts on a regular basis and consistently connecting with readers. In each retelling (and in each rereading), illness identities repeat accepted (and acceptable) images of and responses to depression. Each text becomes a resource for self-evaluation, self-doctoring, and, perhaps, a rhetorical care of the self. Through processes of social interaction, including textual exchanges, we author ourselves using available linguistic and rhetorical tools. These self-narratives deploy recognizable symbols to project the identities that others may then read in our performances. This, then, might begin to explain the popularity of "treatises" on depression: such texts offer expressions and constructions of selves, elaborating for writers and readers the set of codes through which to interpret their own and others' experiences.

As recent work in medical anthropology and narrative medicine demonstrates, stories are rich means for displaying and delimiting the boundaries of illnesses such as depression.[11] Yet too often, stories are considered to be mere reflections of individual experience. To the contrary, they act as powerful coercive devices, sanctioning particular selves and experiences while ignoring others. Depression is a deeply gendered phenomenon, a fact that begins within reports of risk that inform men that they are only half as likely as women to experience or be diagnosed with the illness. But the gendering of depression runs far deeper than this statistic, though the ratio seems to provide objective proof of subjective illness experiences. Men and women inhabit depression differently: they do so, in part, because of the stories that provide them models for social interaction. It is not merely the manifestation of *illness* that the discourse genders, however. It is also the particularities of lives and of selves—in other words, the experiences of *health*—that display the effects of the discourse's gendering. I use *gender* here as a verb to signal the processes through which individuals and experiences become designated as masculine or feminine. Stories of depression—whether literary memoirs or brief anecdotes included to "give life" to news features—describe the contours of such gendered self-authoring. They do this, in part, through standard narratives that serve as the template for acceptable storytelling.

Within the discourse of depression, telling a story that fails to praise bio-medicine risks being dismissed for not recognizing those for whom the pharmaceuticals have provided real cures.[12] A February 2008 *Newsweek* blog reports on a meta-analysis of SSRI drug trial data that concludes the drugs are of little more benefit than placebos for many patients. In response, user comments range from supporting to angrily dismissive, such as this from "MNtoFL": "I must say it's articles like this and nut jobs like Tom Cruise who do so many people a disservice."[13] The anger evident in MNtoFL's comment displays the regulatory force of standard biomedical narratives of depression. Equating analysis of drug trial reports to Cruise's talk show statements against psychiatry may be faulty logic, but the standard narrative of pharmaceutical intervention provides the argumentative warrant for MNtoFL's outrage. Similar standard narratives constrain the possible stories of breast cancer, as Judy Segal's work demonstrates. Her work challenges the common narrative of survival through a refusal to abandon one's children. Segal argues that such a narrative inherently accuses mothers who do not survive of not loving their children enough. One radio talk show host responds to Segal's critique by suggesting Segal needs "a better attitude."[14] Segal her*self* becomes the target of narrative regulation: she should learn how to tell proper stories, the talk show host's reaction implies. Such dismissals provide a powerful disincentive for individuals to narrate the conflicting details of their own experiences. Instead, they rely on stock narratives—of empowering maternal love, of the benefits of pharmaceuticals, of medical compliance—to communicate their experiences.

Standard narratives are necessarily reductive—they offer singular plots that encourage conformity. Segal's response to the radio host originates from her analysis of the particular phrases and linguistic structures that render some women inaudible within the narrative frame in which breast cancer is usually displayed. As a rhetorician, she attends closely to these matters of expression. Similarly, Arthur Frank's work on childhood cancer narratives reveals that popular news media reports "perform a sleight of hand; they make the social context" of particular individuals "disappear."[15] Such reports fall back on stock character and their attitudes (one child's "openness," another's "withdrawal") and elide the contextual surroundings (each child's "history of relationships with other people . . . that produces the different behaviors").[16] Frank's solution to these elisions proposes an ethics of listening that reorganizes the responsibilities of healthy and ill individuals.[17] The former must learn to "hear" and the latter to "express" illness.[18] An ethics based on these "mutual responsibilities" enables the recognition of human frailty *and* human creativity; it enables what I am calling a rhetorical care of the self, which attends to the specifics of life and language. Such an ethics must grapple with the specificity of narratives and discursive patterns in order to open up new patterns of communication.

The Language of Stories of Depression

In the discourse of depression, stories connect individuals with others who have experienced the illness, and, in the process, they offer models against which to evaluate and author the self. For discourse analysts and medical rhetoricians, the general shape of standard illness narratives regulates the stories that may be told, but the details of narrative expression reveal the modes of gendering the illness. As individuals learn to tell their stories within the discourse, they take on the specifically gendered illness identities that are expressed within the standard narratives. To understand stories as more than communicative devices requires analysis on at least two levels: the accumulation of standard narratives enforces particular identities, so attention must be paid to the most common plots and characters; in addition, the specific articulations of individual stories encode a range of acceptable self-performances. The stories told about depression gender its identities at both levels. Women are the most common lead characters within stories of depression, and the roles in which they are portrayed encode a gendered economy of health and illness. In addition, the specific details of women's stories—and those of men suffering from depression—shape both their illness experiences and the responses expected of readers.

In 2005, NIMH published a pamphlet entitled *Stories of Depression: Does This Sound Like You?* The subtitle immediately asks for identification from the reader; the implied action is one of judging the self against the two stories contained in the pamphlet. In the pamphlet, two stories—"Brenda's Story" and "Rob's Story"—describe a series of standard events and experiences. Each story includes descriptions of symptoms; moments of recognition of illness; responses to illness; and resolutions. The specific language in which these events are related, however, reveals significant differences that help differentiate the illness identities along gendered lines. Table 5.1 places the two

TABLE 5.1
"Brenda's" and "Rob's" Stories of Depression

	Brenda's story	Rob's story
Introduction		Things in my life were going all right. I had just gotten my GED and was starting a new job in a week. My family was really proud of me.
Symptoms	It was really hard to get out of bed in the morning. I just wanted to hide under the covers and not talk to anyone. I didn't feel much like eating and I lost a lot of weight. Nothing seemed fun anymore. I was tired all the time, yet I wasn't sleeping well at night. *But I knew that I had to keep going because I've got kids and a job. It just felt so impossible, like nothing was going to change or get better.*	But inside, I was feeling terrible. At first I was feeling sad all the time, even though I had no reason to be. *Then the sadness turned into anger, and I started having fights with my family and friends.* I felt really bad about myself, like I wasn't good enough for anyone. It got so bad that I wished I would go to bed and never wake up.
Recognition	I started missing days from work, and a friend noticed that something wasn't right. *She talked to me about the time that she had been really depressed and had gotten help from her doctor.*	My older brother, who I always looked up to, saw that I wasn't acting like my usual self. *He told me straight out that I seemed depressed and that I should talk to a doctor about it.* I hate going to the doctor. I thought, No way am I going in for this.

Action	*I called my doctor and talked about how I was feeling.* She had me come in for a checkup and gave me the name of a psychiatrist, who is an expert in treating depression. Now, I'm seeing the psychiatrist once a month and taking medicine for depression. I'm also seeing someone else for "talk" therapy, which helps me *learn ways to deal with* this illness in my everyday life.	But after a few weeks, I started having problems at work too. Sometimes I wouldn't show up because I wasn't able to sleep the night before. When I got fired, I knew I had to listen to my brother and get help. *I saw a doctor at the health clinic. He told me I had a common illness called depression and that treatment could help.* So I started to see someone at the clinic each week for "talk" therapy. This treatment helps me *learn to control depression in* my everyday life.
Resolution	Everything didn't get better overnight, but I find myself more able *to enjoy life and my children.*	It has taken some time, but *I'm finally feeling like myself again.*

SOURCE: NIMH, *Stories of Depression: Does This Sound Like You?* (2005), emphasis added.

narratives against each other, highlighting the differences in expression from which readers must make judgments about themselves.

As in many of the examples of stories featuring men with depression, Rob's story begins with an affirmation of his successes: "Things in my life were going all right. I had just gotten my GED and was starting a new job in a week. My family was really proud of me." As part of a formula that seems to make it acceptable for a man to experience depression, a feminized disorder, most male narratives are prefaced with the accomplishments (often physical or economic) of the individual. For women, more often than not, the example begins with the symptoms, or the overwhelming nature of life itself. Brenda's story begins immediately with a description of her illness experience: "It was really hard to get out of bed in the morning. I just wanted to hide under the covers and not talk to anyone. . . . But I knew that I had to keep going because I've got kids and a job. It just felt so impossible, like nothing was going to change or get better." Beyond her description of the illness, Brenda signals her affiliation with family—saying "I've got kids." In Rob's story, his symptoms are quite similar (including "feeling sad all the time"), but his orientation toward his family is solitary and antagonistic: "I started having fights with my family." While Brenda recognizes her social obligations and therefore struggles with her illness *on behalf of* her family, Rob's anger and irritability cause him *to fight with* his family and to deny his illness. These reactions mirror a traditional emotional economy, which Robyn Fivush and Janine Buckner sum up as: "She's Sad; He's Mad."[19]

In each story, there is a point of recognition. In Brenda's case, "a friend noticed that something wasn't right. She talked to me about the time that she had been really depressed and had gotten help from her doctor." Here, the collaborative nature of female friendships seems to be reinforced; it is necessary that the friend, too, has experienced depression. For Rob, however, an older brother (and role model) "told me straight out that I seemed depressed and that I should talk to a doctor about it." For Rob, the recognition of depression does not require reciprocal understanding from his brother; it simply requires a directive. The action of seeking treatment—a necessary part of these stories—is essentially the same in both examples (they each consult a doctor), but through therapy Brenda learns "ways to deal with this illness," while Rob learns "to control depression." Brenda works to *accommodate* the illness, eventually being returned to a socially connected state ("to enjoy life and [her] children"); while Rob *overcomes* the illness and returns to his solitary functioning ("I'm finally feeling like myself again"). In these stories, traditional gender roles are maintained, and the desirable outcomes—connected women, solitary men—are represented as equivalent resolutions. Both Brenda's and Rob's stories are what Arthur Frank calls restitution narratives: they discover their depression, seek treatment, and are restored to functioning.[20] Nevertheless, the specific details and discursive choices within each story reveal differences that contribute to the gendering of depression and to the construction of the expected roles individuals assume. These roles serve as the models through which individuals fashion and maintain their own illness identities.

Within longer stories of depression, similar gendered dynamics recur—characters perform predictably gendered roles, providing evidence both of successful self-fashioning in accordance with discursive pressures (these characters are nonfictional) and of the continued relevance of gender within stories of the illness. Two memoirs—Jeffrey Smith's *Where Roots Reach for Water* (1999) and Tracy Thompson's *The Beast* (1996)—highlight differences between men's and women's illnesses and their caretaking repertoires. Though the specific life events differ, both texts feature the central relationship between the depressed protagonist (Smith and Thompson) and his/her partner. In both stories, the partner plays a significant role in helping the protagonist recover. Yet this content—depression overcome (or at least managed) through the intervention of a partner—finds expression along conventionally gendered lines. In the two memoirs, a culturally accessible vocabulary of emotion helps make the protagonists' partners recognizable.[21]

Smith's partner Lisa appears in his narrative to be an understanding, patient, and gentle partner. Smith writes: "My whole life I had been a blessed man, given into the hands of good and faithful women—my mother, my grandmother, and now Lisa. Women who lived fully in the concrete everyday world, and who were stable, in place wherever they were."[22] These women all perform important roles in Smith's quest for self-knowledge and recovery. In one particularly tense scene, Smith is driving home with Lisa, when his attention drifts and he veers toward the shoulder of the road. Noticing Lisa's startled reaction, Smith immediately becomes angry, pulls the car over, and shouts at her. He recounts her reaction: "Her eyes brimmed with tears. She blinked them back."[23] A few pages later, Smith relates Lisa's response to his outburst: "Lisa turned and looked at me. 'You will be fine,' she said. 'You are learning, I can see it. You don't frighten me, but your frustration comes on so abruptly. Is there any way you can warn me?'"[24] In this scene, Lisa is the calm, accepting partner who helps Smith learn to regulate his emotional responses. She meets his anger with tears and then reassurance for him, focusing her energies on his needs.

By contrast, Thompson's partner, Thomas, seems to use his own rage as a primary means of communication. Thomas forcefully helps Thompson see her illness clearly, both by recommending research and treatment, and by confronting her with her own behavior. She admits that "Thomas could confront me with some truths about myself that nobody else had been able to get me to look at before." Nevertheless, she goes on to say, "He could be brutal about it; I even wondered if he took a sadistic pleasure in pointing out my evasions and inconsistencies."[25] While his interventions clearly help Thompson recognize her illness and seek treatment, Thomas is often unyielding and angry.

Thompson recalls one moment when Thomas's caretaking was "destroyed by his rage. . . . The only target for his anger was me. 'You are a *selfish fucked-up person*,' he would say at such moments."[26] Thomas's anger focuses on his own needs and responds to his partner with accusations about her self, not her illness. For both Smith and Thompson, the social support of a partner proves indispensable for their eventual recoveries, yet their partners offer diametrically opposed forms of support. Indeed, the women in these memoirs—whether healthy or ill—display sadness and accommodation; the men, anger and dominance. Together these displays participate in an economy of emotion that further directs women toward behaviors likely to qualify as depression and men toward behaviors more likely to be viewed as aggression. Expressions of masculine anger or feminine grief provide models against which to imagine the self, and they do so within gendered social and professional spaces.

In news reports about depression, stories are far more concise and limited, but they, too, offer gendered pictures of the illness and responses to it. Reading two reports of the same story side by side, for example, reveals significantly different gender roles in response to a son's suicide. The content of this particular story remains consistent—Donna and Phil Satow started the Jed Foundation after their son committed suicide in college—but the two versions of the story differ significantly in the ways they present the details of the Satows' story. First, a *Blues Buster* article, entitled "Suicide: A Whole New View" (published in May 2003), tells the Satows' story sparingly: "Phil . . . Satow knows a lot about suicide, and he learned it the hard way. He runs the Jed Foundation, named for his son, who committed suicide 'out of the blue' while a student at the University of Arizona in 1998. The foundation has a very clear mission: to dramatically lower the suicide rate on college campuses."[27] Then, a *Newsweek* article entitled "Taking Depression On" (published in August 2004) retells the story in more detail: "Donna Satow of New York City had sent two children to college by the time her third, Jed, went off to the University of Arizona. In 1998, as a sophomore, he committed suicide. Today, Satow and her husband run the Jed Foundation, which helps colleges develop strategies for dealing with depression. She'd like all colleges to screen incoming students for depression, the same way they make sure they've had all their immunizations. Satow advises all parents to ask colleges such things as 'What kind of support do you have in case my youngster gets in trouble?' In a world where families agonize over finding the cushiest dorm room and the perfect meal plan, it's a question that could save a student's life."[28] The second version speaks for Donna, expressing the content of the Satow story through the focalization of a grieving mother. The details of her life that are revealed include the fact that she had already "sent two children to college" by the time Jed leaves for the University of Arizona. Significantly, *she* sent *her* children (Jed is described as "her third") to college; Phil's participation in the family's child-rearing is elided in this version.

Donna's story continues with the dramatic action of Jed's suicide, which is described in an independent sentence. In Phil's story, this event is subordinated as a relative clause. In fact, Phil's own life story is truncated in the first version of the story; his life is replaced by the single salient feature that he "knows a lot about suicide" from having "learned . . . the hard way."

Other differences in the expression of the two narratives continue to pattern gendered identities: Donna's story emphasizes connection and collaboration; Phil's story focuses on information and action. Donna runs the foundation *with* her husband in the *Newsweek* version, but Phil is credited with sole leadership in *Blues Buster*. The mission of the foundation also receives different expression in the two texts: in Donna's story, the foundation "helps colleges develop strategies" and Satow herself "advises all parents to ask colleges" about their support for students' mental health. Here, the foundation—under Donna's leadership—appears supportive and advisory. In the story focused on Phil, however, the foundation has a very clear mission: "to dramatically lower the suicide rate on college campuses." *How* this might be accomplished is irrelevant to Phil's story; his narrative is about responding to suicide with demonstrable action. In these two texts, the expression of the same content offers different models for women and men dealing with the tragedy of suicide. Women—modeling themselves on Donna—are more socially connected and collaborative, offering advice to others; men—in the mold of Phil—take action and prevent future tragedies. Within stories of depression, stock characters and familiar plot lines make illness experiences recognizable, but they also set up expectations for performances of the self. Within my corpus, exemplary individuals represent an important site for rhetorical analysis; they offer insight into the illness identities and gendered behaviors that cue health and illness.

Poster Children and Cultural Luminaries: Exemplary Individuals in Stories of Depression

Individual characters in stories of depression serve as examples against and through which readers learn to judge themselves. Chosen presumably for their representativeness, such "exemplars" portray the recognizable faces of the illness; they become what are colloquially referred to as "poster children." In fact, that phrase itself appears three times in relation to individual exemplars within my collection of public discourse.[29] Examining these instances uncovers significant assumptions about depression sufferers, assumptions that are exaggerated by the voyeuristic attention implied by the phrase itself. Kay Redfield Jamison, a noted psychiatrist and professor of medicine at Johns Hopkins University, suffers from bipolar disorder. She earns the designation of "poster child" by virtue of the popularity of her memoir *An Unquiet Mind* (1997). One article describes this text as "a frighteningly evocative descent into despair," and goes on, in the next phrase, to note that it "sold 300,000 copies and made Jamison something of a celebrity poster child for mental illness."[30] Here, the market success of her memoir makes Jamison not only representative (a poster child), but also famous (a *celebrity* poster child). A sense of Jamison as an object of the public gaze is clear in this article. She is described by her location, "in the tidy study of her Washington, D.C., home," where she "looks up from behind her short pale blond bangs and cites a litany of alarming numbers" about suicide. In setting this particular scene, the article evokes a domestic space ("the tidy study of her . . . home"), and further emphasizes Jamison's physical appearance, noting that she "looks up from behind her short pale blond bangs." Indeed, though she is used in the article as an expert source, her information is "alarming," made more so, perhaps, by its expression through a clearly objectified and gendered subject.

Jamison's celebrity results from the self-revelations within and commercial success of her memoir; Philip Burguieres, on the other hand, "never set out to be the poster child for depression in high places." A successful businessman, indeed "the youngest-ever CEO of a Fortune 500 company," Burguieres "discovered that his presence as a 'player' had . . . power."[31] Unlike Jamison, whose celebrity status emerges from her illness, Burguieres uses power that predates his depression; he accepts the role of "poster child" in order to use the power of his financial and social standing to change perceptions of the illness. Arguably, Jamison's work has been equally directed at reducing stigma and her status is equally powerful (she is a professor at a major research university), but the story that cites her does not make it a point to outline her professional prestige before (or during) her illness. Burguieres's depression seems not to have affected his career (whereas Jamison's illness seems to have defined hers): two years following a severe depressive episode, "Burguieres was still an A-list force on the Houston business and social scene."[32] More, "he found himself richer than ever. For the first time he owned his full humanity."[33] The article applauds Burguieres for "open[ing] a window into a rarefied but closely guarded world" of top business executives who suffer from depression.[34] Indeed, he speaks from his cultural and financial position, and he achieves the "full humanity" afforded through a combination of (restored) health and power.[35] For Burguieres, the poster child role is something he accepts and uses to advance his agenda; for Jamison, the role is assumed to be a part of her identity. Jamison's case is instructive for women: the text does not give her agency within the role of poster child; instead, it objectifies her and subtly negates her power as an expert on and firsthand witness to illness.

Men such as Burguieres may have just cause to be cautious of the title "poster child," and not simply for its clearly infantilizing overtones. In an article featuring Elizabeth Wurtzel, the danger of appearing to seek public attention explains much of Wurtzel's negative publicity. More than Jamison, Wurtzel seems to relish the idea of being a poster child. Her own picture adorns the cover of her memoir, *Prozac Nation*, and her Hollywood double—Christina Ricci—poses unclothed in the cover art for the film made from the book in 2001. It is impossible to avoid the voyeuristic, even pornographic, attention paid both to Wurtzel herself (and her body double Ricci) and to the depressed life so vividly on display in her text. Yet, the danger of such publicity appears to be that it "smacks of self-pity and reeks of marketing research" in the words of a *Dallas Observer* article.[36] Such unflattering opinions are brushed aside, though they are perhaps inadvertently reinforced, in an article entitled "Women Behaving Badly" that appears in *Newsweek* magazine. Calling Wurtzel an "infamous prodigy," the article nevertheless scoffs at the possibility that she "staged a decade of depression so that she could emerge as its poster child."[37]

Yet while defending her from unfair attacks such as those of the *Dallas Observer*, the article nevertheless returns the focus to Wurtzel's physical appearance, something that parallels Burguieres's business successes as a defining characteristic. "Her face is drawn," the article describes, "and long strands of hair have come loose from her untidy blond bun."[38] In instances of exemplary women, blond hair appears to stand in for surprising expertise (as in Jamison's blond bangs) and for emotional disclosure (as in Wurtzel's untidy blond bun). The CEO's hair does not warrant mentioning. Physical details of women's appearances as "poster children" reinforce their status as objects for display within the discourse; they are to be viewed more than they are to be respected. Both Jamison and Wurtzel are defined largely by their illness; they embody it more fully than Burguieres does his, which appears to be an adjunct to his professional life. Neither expertise nor success can be represented without qualification through the lens of gender. These exemplars serve as models for individuals as they author themselves: women must be aware of their physical objectification, and men must attend to their professional standing in order to be recognizable. Another kind of exemplary character in my corpus—the various individuals who function as anecdotal evidence—projects expectations of relationships with medications and alternative therapies.

IN MY CORPUS of news reports, seventy-seven personal stories offer individuals' experiences as examples of depression. Six stories feature girls (up to college age) and eleven feature boys (up to college age); thirty-nine feature women, and twenty-three feature men. Among these stories, the women display an emotional repertoire of worry, anxiety and grief. Men are far more likely to display anger, violence (suicide and/or homicide) and denial. Such stories of depression offer models of acceptable illness behavior for women and men. Drawing on and recirculating a vocabulary that justifies sadness and emotional volatility in women and anger and hostility in men, such stories form the basis for constructing individual illness identities. This emotional economy evokes gendered responses from critical reviews of depression memoirs. A sampling of reviews of five memoirs written by women and five composed by men reveals a public preference for emotional disclosures from women and for more objective accounts from men. Memoirs by women are praised for their authentic emotional revelations: Danquah is credited with "discuss[ing] movingly how she overcame depression" and "tell[ing] her story poignantly and affectingly."[39] Martha Manning's *Undercurrents* depicts "events . . . sensitively and insightfully."[40] And, in *Prozac Diary*, Slater "movingly, even poetically, grapples" with her illness and its cure.[41] Beyond such praise for emotional struggle and display, *The National Review* describes Wurtzel, author of *Prozac Nation*, as "a more zaftig version of Kate Moss," emphasizing the author's physical appearance and drawing the self (as author) into the evaluation of the text.[42] In the reviews of each of these memoirs written by women, stories are evaluated for their sensitivity to nuanced emotional experiences.

Memoirs written by men, on the other hand, receive praise for their objective collection of information and criticism for overly sentimental revelations. Wolpert's *Malignant Sadness* offers "solace and useful information"[43] and Smith "is learned and thoughtful" in his *Where Roots Reach for Water*, even though the reviewer "did not find the narrative very gripping."[44] If such reviews may be seen as lessons in how readers should approach these texts and how sufferers should take on the illness identities portrayed in them, a picture of depression as a gendered phenomenon begins to come into focus. Andrew Solomon's text is praised for its comprehensive nature, but he himself is criticized for "charting [his] own battles in sometimes greater detail than one needs."[45] Emotion and vivid expression receive praise when authors are women; information, objectivity, and comprehensiveness are valued when authors are men. Stories of depression thus take shape within a set of gendered expectations for their kind and content. Individuals must craft their stories in response to those already circulating, but they must also conform to the gender roles expected of them: women display greater emotionality; men, rationality.

In the discourse of depression, women come to be characterized by their depressions—it is the first thing we often learn about them—and depression itself inhabits female form. In one article, "Depression . . . wears a human face—the face of Mary Jo West."[46] Men, on the other hand, are likely to be only secondarily associated with their depressions, and that association usually occurs after a more prestigious identity has already been established. For example, "William Styron, Mike Wallace, Art Buchwald, cultural luminaries with one trait in common: All are prominent men who have publicly revealed that they suffer from depression."[47] In these opposing instances, the men are "prominent" and "cultural luminaries" who also suffer from depression; West, even though she is a pioneering journalist and accomplished individual, is described as the mask—the "human face"—of depression. Indeed, when women are given identities that precede their illness identities, they are often pictured in domestic, familial scenes. In 1995, when Colin Powell was considering a bid for the presidency, his wife's depression became newsworthy. As an exemplar, Alma Powell is first described by her domestic affiliation: "By all accounts, Alma Powell, 57, is a strong and loving wife."[48] Though she is later in the article given credit for her own public successes, her initial introduction is as a wife, and the description of her as both "strong and loving" suggests the cultural value placed upon women's emotional labor, especially when we compare her identity to the cultural and economic status afforded Styron, Wallace, Buchwald, and the CEO poster child, Burguieres. While the content of depression stories often remains consistent, the expression of individual stories encourages attention to women's physical and emotional displays and to men's economic and cultural successes.

Women's participation within narratives of depression often place them within domestic social networks. But when they are depressed, women seem to be isolated from those networks; they are left without the support structures they routinely provide for others. In a section of *Depression: What Every Woman Should Know*, titled "The Path to Healing," treatment becomes "a partnership between the patient and the health care provider."[49] Suggesting that women must first recognize "the signs of depression," and then "be evaluated by a qualified professional," the section avoids mentioning any role for family and friends in the healing process.[50] By contrast, *Men and Depression* contains a section that encourages the same steps—recognition and treatment—but places those activities within a social network. Immediately assuming that, in the words of the section's title, family and friends can help, the men's text writes that "the most important thing anyone can do for a man who may have depression is to help him get to a doctor."[51] To do this, the text recommends "talk[ing] to him" about depression, "help[ing] him understand that depression . . . is nothing to be ashamed about."[52] The section goes on to suggest that "you may need to make an appointment for the depressed person and accompany him to the doctor."[53] Unlike the second-person address in the women's booklet, where "you" refers to the sufferer (who owes it to herself and her family to seek help), this "you" is clearly a reader *other* than the sufferer. The men's booklet clearly anticipates readers who are also caretakers, whereas the women's booklet seems to place responsibility on the depressed woman alone.

The caretaking suggested as necessary for men goes beyond encouraging his initial diagnosis in *Men and Depression*. Once he begins to receive treatment, the booklet explains, family and friends should monitor his medication and attendance at therapy sessions, encourage him to be honest about drug and alcohol use, and continue to offer emotional support. For women, however, the path to healing is more solitary. A checklist offers similar steps as a series of imperative statements: check your symptoms, talk to a health professional, choose a treatment approach, and be an informed consumer. "Along with professional treatment," the section sums up for its female readers, "there are a number of other things you can do to help yourself get better."[54] Alone. Depressed women—whose symptoms may be indistinguishable from ordinary and expected emotional turmoil—are assumed to be their own caretakers. Depressed men, on the other hand, are encouraged to admit that their emotional symptoms are the result of a "real" illness, but they are also supported by a wider array of family and friends who will collaborate with them on treatment.

Stories about depression establish gendered dynamics of illness—angry, stoic men, and tearful, emotional women—and of treatment: networked caretaking for men, solitary self-help for women. Such dynamics inform the plot lines and the speaking roles available within the discourse. When they are in caretaking positions, women (wives and mothers) are given voice through direct quotation, particularly when they are speaking for a son's illness. Among the eleven news stories featuring boys, five include quotations from the boys' mothers that assess, diagnose, or describe their sons' illnesses. In a sixth narrative, both parents are present, but only the mother is directly quoted. More significantly, these mothers have their "hearts . . . broken again and again";[55] they "worry when a trip" doesn't alleviate a child's "inexplicable bleakness";[56] they embark "on long search[es] to find help";[57] they see "signs of . . . behavioral and emotional problems."[58] Such diligent and constant care—attributed to mothers of depressed sons—stands in stark contrast to the institutional and self-care displayed in narratives about girls who are depressed.

In two of the brief stories about young girls who are depressed, it is not a parent but rather a doctor who introduces, diagnoses, and explains the girl's illness. For example, "Dr. Fassler recalls the case of Caroline, who, as a 4-year-old preschooler, was a smart, serious, quiet child who kept largely to herself. . . . Then, without a word of warning to anyone . . . Caroline walked into the middle of a busy four-lane highway."[59] The shock of Caroline's actions "without a word of warning" might suggest either that she was more secretive than the boys whose behavior receives so much attention, or that girls, assumed to be more verbal than boys, do not merit the same scrutiny for nonverbal signs of illness. This latter reading seems to be reinforced by the level of attention to behavior in stories of boys who are depressed. For example, "Barbara Sheldon's son never napped as an infant, was actually running when he was seven months old and insisted on trying to play in the oven as a toddler,"[60] and "Lorna Grivois . . . said she had seen signs of her son's behavior and emotional problems when he was a baby."[61] Girls, by contrast, seem to become depressed without physical warning signs: "Brianne Camilleri had it all: two involved parents, a caring older brother and a comfortable home near Boston. But that didn't stop the overwhelming sense of hopelessness that enveloped her in ninth grade."[62] In these descriptions, boys' behavior is carefully monitored and detailed, whereas girls' depressed behavior appears inexplicable to parents and doctors. That young girls could become depressed "without a word of warning" seems to run counter to the illness identity—a verbal, emotional display—prescribed for them. It is almost as if they are expected already to self-monitor and self-regulate, while their male counterparts receive discursive scrutiny and descriptive attention.

As girls become women, their experiences with depression come to be tied explicitly to domestic and familiar spaces. Tipper Gore's depression mirrors her own mother's struggles with the illness, which "cast a gloomy pall on the household."[63] For Melanie Stokes, a forty-one-year-old mother who "jumped to her death . . . just three months after giving birth to a much-wanted baby girl," the solution, according to her own mother, ought to have included a hospital stay "in cheerful rooms" away from her daughter's troubled domestic space.[64] For several women, the prospect of sending children off to college represents a potential "empty nest" depression. In one article, "Sarah Ripp began pining over the prospect that her daughter, Emily, was going away to college" so much that "her husband has taken to calling her 'the weeping willow.'"[65] As painful as these circumstances must be, the danger represented is not necessarily illness for the individual woman, but the loss of a mother's caretaking for an entire family. A woman's illness threatens her children; for example, "Linda Meyer, 41, recalls how helpless her husband felt when she was stricken by overwhelming anxiety and irritability after the births of their daughters, now 8 and 11. 'He just was dumbfounded,' she says. 'He had no idea what he could do to make me better.' But when a mother is depressed over the long term, it is usually the children who suffer most. 'If you can't take pleasure in anything, that is very crushing for a child,' says Berger. 'What children need to thrive is the twinkle in the mother's eye. And that is what depression robs the mother of.'"[66] Indeed, the same article goes on to cite a medical ethicist who claims that "doctors may want to recommend that women with severe PPD [postpartum depression] limit their family size." The solution to women's depression is, here, to limit her family size, suggesting that her own path to healing is less important than her duty to protect her family. Children, in this vignette, "need . . . the twinkle in the mother's eye," and in its absence, fathers are "just . . . dumbfounded." Ripp's husband may call her "the weeping willow," but his caretaking responsibility does not appear to include any other response to his wife's illness.

When men are depressed, however, they receive more supporting and constructive responses from their social networks. For one physician who became depressed, help came from "see[ing] himself through the eyes of his wife and children."[67] In another story, a depressed man's mother lies "awake in bed, listening to her 32-year-old son pacing his room."[68] Such social support from wives and mothers, when withdrawn, seems to lead to male violence. For example, "William Sennit . . . told friends that he planned to kill Melody Arons . . . and himself after she broke off their five-year relationship."[69] In men's stories, a network of domestic caretaking appears to monitor and respond to their depressions. Within the discourse of depression, much attention is paid to the potentially volatile emotions of healthy women. When they become ill, however, they are subject largely to medical attention. For men, whose emotional range is assumed to be much more stable, a lot of attention, particularly from the women in their lives, focuses on them once they become ill. The stoic, solitary male receives careful monitoring when he inhabits a depressed illness identity.

The often overly emotional woman, by contrast, is monitored *before* she is recognized as ill and then is offered little discursive support and a fair amount of criticism (for being a bad mother, for example) until she can resume a healthy identity. The complex, shifting economies of caretaking and social support shape depression as an illness that women are susceptible to, but also that they have primary caretaking responsibility for. Within these storylines, women and men must negotiate their senses of self and learn to practice forms of self- and other-doctoring. In my interviews with women experiencing symptoms of depression, these emotional economies were very much present and persuasive factors in the women's conversations. This fact demonstrates the power of standard characters and storylines to reinforce gendered health and illness identities.

Constructing the Pharmaceutical Woman

At the turn of the twenty-first century, the self is increasingly understood in chemical terms, and practices of self-doctoring respond in kind. Emily Martin describes the contemporary construction of the self alongside and through drugs with the phrase "pharmaceutical person."[70] In doing so, she calls attention to the relationships between individuals and the medications they ingest. When drugs have "personalities"—evidenced by the marketing campaigns that introduce them to us—and when we are not "ourselves" without them, notions of personhood confuse the *self* and the medications it ingests. In the discourse of depression, the "pharmaceutical person" incorporates both psychopharmacological agents (Prozac, Zoloft) and also more "natural" supplements such as Saint-Johnswort, an herbal treatment for the illness, as physical means of self-doctoring. Within my corpus, stories about the "pharmaceutical person" are most detailed when they display women's practices of self-doctoring.[71]

One such story—the lead in a *Newsweek* article on Saint-Johnswort—offers a restitution narrative that displays a simple progression from illness back to health. In this case, the curative agent is not a sanctioned psychopharmaceutical, but rather an herbal supplement. The article narrates Karin Taylor's illness and recovery:

> Karin Taylor's black moods were often accompanied by inexplicable bouts of insomnia, crying and lethargy. By last summer she'd sunk so low she didn't care if she lived or died. But Taylor balked when her physician suggested a common antidepressant: she didn't feel comfortable taking drugs. Fortunately, she says, a friend visiting from California suggested a natural herb called Saint Johns wort. Within three weeks, Taylor's depression had lifted. 'I feel restored,' says the 58-year-old Toronto accountant, who continues to take two herb capsules daily. 'I'm my normal self again.'[72]

Taylor's attitude toward pharmaceutical treatment—she "didn't feel comfortable taking drugs"—is represented in opposition to the bleak details of her illness. Not caring to live, Taylor is still "not comfortable" with the antidepressant medications suggested by her doctor; she "balks" at the suggestion. Instead of following the established medical advice, Taylor prefers her own expertise, and that of her friend, who suggests "a natural herb." The contrast between "drugs" and "herbs" is a common and, to some extent, false distinction within the discourse of depression. Suspicion of the synthetic production of drugs is not paralleled by suspicion of the processing of "natural" supplements, though both could be understood as manufacturing processes. Taylor "continues to take two herb capsules daily," an action of self-doctoring that appears unproblematic and even central to her personal identity.

The conclusion to the article returns to the biomedical ethos of pharmaceutical treatment for depression. It judges, albeit mildly, individuals such as Taylor who choose "natural" supplements over biomedicine. The article concludes: "Further research is clearly needed. . . . Meanwhile, America's penchant for self-care ensures that remedies like Saint-Johnswort will continue to flourish."[73] The phrase "penchant for self-care" interprets practices of self-doctoring with herbal medications as mildly indulgent, if basically harmless. A "remedy" such as Saint-Johnswort might be nonstandard, but it will "flourish" thanks to the successes reported by individuals such as Taylor. Placing individual stories in the context of biomedical research ("more" of which "is needed"), the article encourages readers to show allegiance to institutional medicine, even as the allure of a successful "natural" remedy clearly appeals to them. The tension between the biomedical and the natural pharmaceutical person does not resolve in this or other narratives within my corpus. Instead, readers are shown a variety of conflicting orientations toward health and illness, but all orientations reinforce necessary self-modification primarily through pharmaceutical or other medicinal compounds.

In the act of reading, the audience adopts a variety of stances toward the self, but in the end, all such stances site responsibility for maintaining health with the individual alone. Various drug therapies may cause depression to lift, but the articulation of the self is an individual responsibility. In Taylor's story, cure (via Saint-Johnswort) appears in the passive voice and off stage. The narrative focuses on Taylor's own self-doctoring: Taylor's direct quotations assert her restoration but do not detail her treatment regimen, which is naturalized through third-person narration. Instead, her voice is used to validate a whole range of practices—including the antidepressants at which she "balked"— because return to a "normal self" is the primary focus of the story. Accepting Taylor's story entails valuing her self-doctoring: asserting the individual's responsibility to take action on herself in the face of depression.

In other narratives, women's self-doctoring choices are represented within expressions of their gendered identities. An anonymous woman's experiences with "B vitamins" as a cure for her depression are couched in a private, domestic setting:

> She was making lunch for herself and a friend one Saturday this spring when an unfamiliar feeling swept over her. The 50-year-old social worker had fallen deep into depression two years earlier, and had given up on prescription antidepressants when the first one she tried left her sluggish, sexually dormant and numb to her own emotions. Then, in mid-March, she heard about a naturally occurring substance called SAMe (pronounced Sammy). She had been taking it for just a few days when she began setting the table that Saturday morning. A ginger-miso sauce was chilling in the fridge, and she was garnishing her finest plates with fresh anemones. Suddenly, there it was: a sense of undiluted pleasure.[74]

The nearly miraculous return of "undiluted pleasure" occurs within the context of lunchtime preparations for this woman: she is "setting the table," "garnishing her finest plates," and a "ginger-miso sauce [is] chilling in the fridge." She is, in other words, the perfect homemaker preparing for a visit with her friend. The effects of the natural supplement within this story suggest that *cure* returns women to a domestic scene from which *illness* has somehow alienated them. The article does not pass judgment—as it did in the case of Saint-Johnswort—on this particular practice of self-doctoring. Instead, it speaks as the voice for such alternative therapies. "In other words," the article concludes, "many of us could arm ourselves against low moods, bad joints and weak hearts simply by upping our intake of B vitamins. That may sound less exciting than taking a miracle supplement. But with luck, it could keep you from ever needing one."[75] The danger here, it seems, is for individuals who refuse the form of self-doctoring, for those who do not "up their intake," and are therefore not doing enough to avoid future pharmaceutical intervention. The shift from first-person plural ("many of us") to second-person ("it could keep you") further reinforces the directive message of this text. In both stories, the pharmaceutical person is not the longtime user of Prozac, but an average woman who is searching for relief from symptoms and a return to her "normal" life. She is embedded in her domestic and social scenes; she discreetly hides her illness and even, to some extent, its cure behind the descriptions of her gendered display of health. These exemplars of depression participate in the discourse's larger pattern of gendered economies of health and illness, productivity and caretaking. Such economies reflect larger cultural assumptions about gender, but they are also shaped and reiterated within stories of depression, helping to stage gendered performances of health and illness.

"You Know": Assumed Plots and Restricted Actions

Stories of depression situate readers in relation to their gendered selves as they experience mental health and illness. Some evidence drawn from my corpus and my interviews offers insight into the ways that individuals take up and use the available illness identities. Conversations among women experiencing symptoms of depression, as well as a question and answer section included in *Blues Buster*, display practices of self-doctoring that implicate women in the construction of their own gendered illness identities. The pharmaceutical person, the emotional economy of health and illness, and the gendering of social networks are all tools with which individuals may define their health and illness identities. In some cases, these tools form the means of tactical responses to the discourse of biological psychiatry, but more often they appear to be taken up according to the dictates of the discursive strategy, as practices of self-doctoring.

In one interview, the women seem to work toward a version of the pharmaceutical person. Su-Ting begins by telling the story of a relative who was hospitalized for an unspecified form of depression:

SU: Yeah because one of my relatives are diagnosed [with] depression or bipolar or, yeah I don't know what the diagnosis [is]. But I know she was hospitalized. So I don't like to use the word "depression" to express this feeling [of mine], because I think people must be insane or need to take some medicine, yeah.

CLAIRE: Yeah, that's what my mom says.

TIFF: Mmm hmm.

CLAIRE: When I tried telling her [that] I really wanted help, I wanted a friend to talk to . . . she's like, "It's a mental issue, Claire," and . . . "Why can't you just fix it yourself?" she acted like. "It's all in your head," she said. But I didn't think that that was the case [breathes out].

SU: Then maybe medication can help? I don't mean you should try [it] . . . I just say it's . . . if that could help.

CLAIRE: Yeah, if it's you've like a chemical imbalance.

TIFF: But sometimes it's not.

CLAIRE: Yeah, well, I don't know how you know unless you try the medication and it works or something.

Su-Ting first admits that she associates the term *depression* with a severe condition, and she therefore rejects it as a label for herself. Claire responds by saying that her own mother might agree with this assessment (thinking Claire herself is not depressed, but rather just suffering from "a mental issue"). Claire goes on, however, to suggest that she and her mother do not share orientations toward this issue. Claire would like "a friend to talk to" and her mother wants her to "fix it" herself. This painful revelation for Claire—she speaks very softly and hesitantly at this point in the interview—is met by Su-Ting's suggestion that medication might be necessary. Neither the women in the interview nor Claire's mother have taken her request for "a friend to talk to" seriously: for Su-Ting, the solution might be drugs; for Claire's mother, it is a matter of willpower. Nevertheless, Tiffany expresses the collective anxiety about medications for depression when she responds to Claire's statement that a "chemical imbalance" might be helped by such drugs. "But sometimes it's not" a chemical imbalance, Tiffany asserts, providing a chance for a more critical engagement with this model for depression. Unfortunately, however, the women do not take this opportunity to consider what other models for depression might exist. Claire's final turn suggests a capitulation to simply *trying* medication to see if it might work. This conversation displays the discursive pressure toward self-medicating; it provides a snapshot of women potentially accepting a pharmaceutical identity when no other stories are available as models.

Another possible location for critical engagement with the discourse occurs within a question-and-answer column that appears on the back page of each *Blues Buster* newsletter. In this section, entitled "Managing Your Mood," Michael Yapko takes questions from readers and responds to them. The questions often seem to model themselves on standard depression narratives; Yapko's responses offer both potential sites for a tactical critique of those narratives, and also reiterations of coercive strategies that require self-doctoring. In one issue, a woman seeks advice about a depression that she identifies as relating to her emotional dependence on her children. She writes:

I am a married middle-age university professor and technician who is dealing with ever-increasing depression. I have been tested and found to have a slight adult attention-deficit problem. I am an only child, and my late father was an alcoholic. I am really having an "empty nest" problem as my two children are growing up and my son soon will be leaving home for college. Somehow I am too emotionally dependent on them. I am taking 20–30 mg of Adderall daily for the ADD. It improves not only my mental focus but my mood as well. Also, I take SAM-e for depression, and it seems to make a steady improvement in mood. Sometimes, I wonder if I am not bipolar as my moods can change very rapidly. Do you have any suggestions for additional medication or therapy?[76]

The question displays a complex array of self-doctoring practices: submitting the self to testing, ingesting a variety of medications, judging the self against emotional expectations, and seeking additional medical advice. Each of these practices is also narratively embedded, shaped by common stories of depression. First, the woman feels "too emotionally dependent" on her children—signaling not only that she defines much of her health in relation to her family, but also that she is struggling with the role of caretaker for her children. Then, she lists a number of pharmaceutical treatments that she uses to improve her "mental focus" and "mood." In this letter, the woman fails to question any of the conflicting stories she tells about herself.

In his response to this inquiry, Yapko focuses attention on the woman's use of various drugs, suggesting that she has too quickly taken on the identity of a pharmaceutical person. He writes: "Your letter poses some interesting issues, especially in light of two obvious contradictions. First, you say that SAM-e creates a 'steady improvement' of your mood, but in your very first sentence you say you are dealing with 'ever increasing depression.' Second, you declare your problem to be an 'empty nest' issue because you are 'too emotionally dependent' on your children, yet you focus treatment on changing your body chemistry."[77] Yapko's comments note the contradictions in the woman's self-description, and they highlight the ways in which her identity has been shaped by the emotional and pharmaceutical examples that surround her. She has constructed what to her seems a coherent illness identity but to Yapko appears to be an incomplete collection of conflicting discourses.

In another issue, Yapko's response demonstrates the difficulty for women to be seen outside of their familial roles and responsibilities. A woman writes, describing herself as "a psychologist with a family history of depression."[78] In her question, she describes her concern for her brother who she fears "is currently overmedicated," and asks for advice on "approach[ing] the doctor so that family members can be included in the [treatment] team."[79] Although she has explicitly described her professional credentials (as a psychologist), Yapko's response begins by referring to her as "an extraordinary sister."[80] After her sibling role is thus reestablished, Yapko goes on to caution that the "doctor has no obligation to anyone other than the patient." Essentially, he says, the sister cannot expect to be included in the treatment—despite the fact that her caretaking makes her "extraordinary." The woman is divested of her professional expertise and returned to the role of caring sister. Yapko's response ignores entirely the woman's request for discursive strategies for approaching her brother's doctor. In this instance, his response participates in the larger discursive strategy of reinforcing gendered caretaking roles and responsibilities. The woman's question, however, offers an important tactical challenge to these strategies: she asks for rhetorical tools for promoting her brother's self-care.

Yapko's advice, however, often reiterates gendered roles in relation to depression. In two parallel questions, a wife and a husband write to Yapko about their depressed spouses. In the first text, the woman writes: "My husband is suffering with what seems to be depression." She goes on to describe his symptoms in diagnostic terms (he "doesn't do the things he used to enjoy") and confesses that she does not "know how to help him."[81] Yapko interprets this question as one about *why* the husband has not sought help, ignoring the woman's request for practical strategies. Yapko writes that "[t]here is no easy answer to this question, and many reasons why people don't get the help they need."[82] He continues to pose rhetorical questions such as: "How far are you willing to go to get your family member some help? And at what point do you intervene?"[83] These responses suggest no definitive action for the woman, but Yapko's conclusion clearly acknowledges the wife's responsibility for helping her husband. He writes: "The importance of overcoming the helplessness and initiating an active approach to self-care cannot be overstated. *So keep trying until you find a way.* Bear in mind, though, you can't force someone into voluntary treatment."[84] Here, the woman's mastery of diagnostic terminology is irrelevant and her caretaking responsibilities are assumed but not enumerated.

For a distressed husband, however, a far less coherent description of his wife's illness elicits specific strategies for response. The husband writes: "I love my wife, but she's driving me crazy. She's been going through her own personal hell for the last few months with depression. She's in therapy and on medications. I'd love to be able to help her, but I don't know what to do. I don't want to baby her, but I also don't want to push her too much. How do I handle a depressed family member?"[85] Yapko's response is far more definitive for this husband than it was for the wife who has essentially the same question. Yapko starts by suggesting that the husband ought to handle his wife "compassionately, lovingly and firmly."[86] The column continues with a series of tips—written as bullet-point commands—that offer concrete action. Here, the advice offers more straightforward guidance, suggesting a response to the husband's displayed lack of control in the situation. Where the wife in the first text describes depression in familiar symptomatic terms, the husband in the second confesses only that his wife is "driving [him] crazy." Clearly, the emotional economy represented within the stories of depression operates within these two homes: the woman offers symptom monitoring and continued caretaking; the man feels overwhelmed by his wife's illness.

Similarly, for the women I interviewed, depression is a gendered illness, but their discussion of this gendering reveals more about normal emotional economies than it does about the illness itself. In one interview, Tiffany responds to my question about whether depression is a gendered phenomenon by introducing examples of men whom she suspects or knows to be depressed. She concludes her turn with the statement that men are more likely to hide their depression, and the other women collaborate on this gendering of emotions:

CLAIRE: You know women are more sensitive too=

TIFF: =yeah that's true, women are *definitely* more sensitive.

KE: What do you mean by that?

TIFF: They're more willing to show it. I mean they're more willing to like, like *feel* the feeling you know what I mean? Like, *be* the feeling [laughs] . . .

CLAIRE: Well, I . . . was only talking about feelings, (about gender and) women usually want to talk about it more.

PAIGE: I think women don't, I think men feel things too; but, I think an emotional life is really important for women. And most women have really *rich* emotional lives. But I think that's not the case for most men. I think that men's lives are rich in other ways, so that sometimes causes a conflict when men and women get together.

In an echo of the NIMH pamphlet's attention to the "fullness" of women's emotional lives, all of the participants seem to agree that women are "more sensitive" and more invested in their "rich emotional lives." Claire begins to answer my question about the potential gendering of depression with the idea that "women are more sensitive," which is immediately reinforced by Tiffany's latching agreement and further emphasis on women's sensitivity. Paige offers her theory of the importance of "an emotional life" to women, even going so far as to suggest that women and men have difficulty relating to each other because of the differences in their commitment to their emotions. In this exchange, the women develop a definition of women's lives as full of emotional complexity. Indeed, for Tiffany, women can be *equated with* their emotions. Here, the commonplace notion of women's greater emotional range and verbal expression of their feelings is clearly taken up by the women. Surrounded by cultural narratives and a vocabulary of emotion that makes these images available, the women define themselves, and their potential illness identities, through the lenses of gender and emotion.

Within the stories of depression, women are portrayed as more emotional than men; for Tiffany, Claire, and Paige, this is a commonsensical notion.

Within the stories of depression, social networks feature women in domestic scenes, coordinating both illness and recovery for themselves and for their families; for the readers of *Blues Buster*, these networks hold true. If storytelling is an ethical act that promotes connection and even healing, then the forms of narrative available are important sites for rhetorical analysis. Within the discourse of depression, narratives set up images of men and women and their life experiences that predispose them (women) to illness or protect them (men) from it. Individuals learn how to be healthy and ill by reading and writing such stories.

IN CONVERSATION rarely do we reiterate information that we assume to be common knowledge. Such common knowledge is often signaled in conversation by the discourse marker "you know" (sometimes articulated in the truncated form "y'know"). According to Deborah Schiffrin, *y'know* functions as a "marker of metaknowledge about what speaker and hearer share . . . [or] about what is generally known."[87] The women who spoke with me about their experiences with symptoms of depression used this discourse marker at key moments to signal common knowledge about social roles and expectations. In effect, "you know" normalizes the stories and subjectivities these women are struggling to adopt and/or reject. Jennifer describes her awareness of depressive symptoms within her work life. She says: "In work environments, I've always gotten along well with people. . . . Usually, I'm a relatively patient person, but I've noticed that I'm not patient with certain people . . . and I don't like that feeling of being short with them and angry at work, and just going home at the end of the day and just, *you know*. It's really bothering me." In this anecdote, Jennifer seeks affirmation as well as asserts common knowledge about depression—her "you know" signals an acceptance of the social obligations her workplace entails and a self-diagnosis of depression for failing to meet those expectations. The social identities available to women restrict behavior and enforce self-doctoring when those behaviors are difficult to enact. Jennifer and her peers collectively understand depression to exist in failed performances of the self—a normally patient person who gets angry at work, or someone who, in Mei's words, "*you know*, [is] not good enough friends with these people." In both cases, the conversational "you know" asserts common knowledge but it also affords an opportunity to interrogate that knowledge.

Self-diagnosis leads to self-help, both of which make use of the available illness (and health) identities in the discourse of depression. As the interview conversation unfolds around types of depression the women have experienced, I ask them what role friends have in relation to these feelings. Social connections, according to Stephanie and Mei, are incredibly important because they have the power to "make [depressive feelings] go away," according to Stephanie. For Mei, this leads to the conclusion that "you just need to keep doing different things so that, *you know*, it helps." Here, "you know" establishes a social imperative for Mei and her peers. They risk being negligent, bringing on their own illness, if they do not perform (socially) as expected. The stories these women tell reinforce gendered encounters with the world and threaten consequences, mainly illness, for failing to engage as expected. Within the discourse of depression, stories function coercively to dictate behavior by representing standard plots, portraying exemplary characters, and modulating the rhetorical treatment of individual subjects. Nevertheless, these stories also offer evidence of tactical resistance to accepting illness identity.

In one interview, Jennifer, Mei, and Stephanie discuss the power of *talk* as a response to their depressive symptoms. Jennifer describes her desire to speak with a doctor; Stephanie relates a story involving a friend's dialogical intervention. Jennifer speaks first:

JENN: I don't know, I think my reasons for seeing a doctor are more for the problems or issues that I have, that I just need some clarification on, and a different perspective. Or, somehow working on my attitude to make me feel better and be more positive about things, instead of so negative.

MEI: But see, I don't know how a doctor is going to help me with that . . . I mean if I'm so aware of what I'm doing then I need to, then I know what I need to do . . .

JENN: I think I need to hear . . . reassurance, because it's like maybe I have the solutions and I've thought about them, but I haven't—I just don't actively do them, because I just want somebody else to tell me that it's okay. That this is, you know, what you should do. This is the path you should take instead of, you know, I might have three different paths and I'm just not sure which one, you know . . . it's the decisions in life that you make and you want to make sure that you make the right ones, um, and not have any regrets, so, yeah=

MEI: =so you, you think of him as like a professional? And you trust his advice, or his opinions?

Here, Jennifer uses "you know" to help the others understand her desire to speak with a doctor. Mei's initial response participates in the self-help narrative: just do it yourself. In response, Jennifer points out how difficult that can be without dialogue. Mei's next response pushes Jennifer to question her faith in a medical professional. Jennifer responds:

JENN: [Well, maybe] I mean, of course you have to put a little rationale in there, that they make sense. . . . Just recently I went to [the campus health center] and . . . I don't know if she was a doctor or a nurse practitioner, but she said something that was contradictory to all the things that I've read and heard and spoken [about] with other doctors. So, you know, you always have to make sure that, yeah, I don't know. I've just come to the point where my thinking I'm not trusting it and it may be skewed and I need, I'm not able to be, an outside perspective. Like I have an outside perspective to help a friend, but I don't have enough outside perspective to help myself, because I'm so involved in it.

MEI: That's true.

JENN: I just can't think clearly, you know? Because I'm biased [laughs], yeah, and you, you have to ask yourself the hard questions and maybe I'm not willing to ask myself the hard questions and someone else can ask me the hard questions to help me decide what to do.

Jennifer's response highlights the power of dialogue—she may not be "willing to ask [herself] the hard questions," but she recognizes the power those questions have of opening up new directions for her. For Stephanie, a friend challenges her self-perception and helps her think about herself as much as her symptoms of illness:

STEPH: My friend said something to me that was very useful, she's the one that, that takes the Zoloft and is, um, suffers from depression too. She said, you know, you're too hard on yourself. The reason you're depressed is that you're too hard on yourself, and I, I stepped back from that and I've been thinking about it for *months*, I mean she said that, I don't know, six months ago, I'm still thinking about it. She's right.

For both Stephanie and Jennifer, dialogue represents a possibly valuable intervention into their experiences. While their stories and those of their peers reflect stereotypical assumptions about women's and men's emotional lives, they are also, at times, willing to question each other about those stories. This, it seems to me, offers a faint promise for a rhetorical self-care. Bringing standard narratives into conversation not as exemplars, but as objects of analysis has at least the potential to open new spaces for self-articulation. Nevertheless, as Segal's cautionary tale about challenging breast cancer narratives suggest, such critiques rarely find supportive conversational partners. Perhaps, then, we should find ways to open up the moments of assumed consensus—to challenge the "you know" in each story as it gets told. One place to start such questioning is the now-ubiquitous and rarely challenged self-diagnostic quiz for depression. This tool, more than any other discursive representation of depression, has become a primary means of self-doctoring. Individuals who have been shaped by the discourse's imprecise definitions, isolating metaphors, and standard stories of gendered emotionality turn quite uncritically to these checklist-style worksheets for help. They submit themselves to the discourse as a first step toward acquiring the illness identity it prescribes.

6

Diagnostic Genres and the
Reconfiguring of Medical Expertise

A 1991 *New Yorker* cartoon by Stephanie Skalisky depicts the *Mona Lisa* as the portrait of a new medical diagnosis (figure 9). Surrounding the image of the painting, block text commands: "Know the four warning signs of Monanucleosis," with contrasting white-on-black lettering that emphasizes the number (four) of symptoms and the name (Monanucleosis) of the disease. Overlaid on the image are text bubbles enumerating each of the signs of illness: "loss of eyebrows and eyelashes" attaches to the corner of an eye; "ever-present enigmatic smile" to the mouth; "rigid posture" gestures to the figure's left arm; and "loss of body parts from the waist down" directs attention into *Mona Lisa*'s lap, beyond the bottom of the frame. Transforming this cultural artifact into a rubric for self-diagnosis, Skalisky's cartoon exaggerates a contemporary obsession with monitoring and, in the process, atomizing the self. Parodying the logic of personal vigilance that promises early detection and cure of illness, the cartoon pokes fun at the expansive scope of medical authority and at an increasingly medicalized attention to our own and others' physical and emotional bodies. In the cartoon, the reader is exhorted to "know the four warning signs" of the illness and, presumably, to act accordingly. The attendant discursive practices of self-doctoring—for example, tallying the presence and absence of items from a standard menu—encourage a view of the self that categorizes otherwise normal experiences and individual features of our own and others' portraits as symptoms of illness. The warning signs of Monanucleosis serve as a comedic example of an increasingly familiar genre, one that appears in pharmaceutical advertising campaigns, patient information brochures, and questionnaires doctors ask patients to complete during routine visits, namely, the symptoms list. This genre offers what appears to be a chance for individuals to practice self-care, guiding them through a series of questions and encouraging consultation and further discussion. Unfortunately, upon closer examination, the

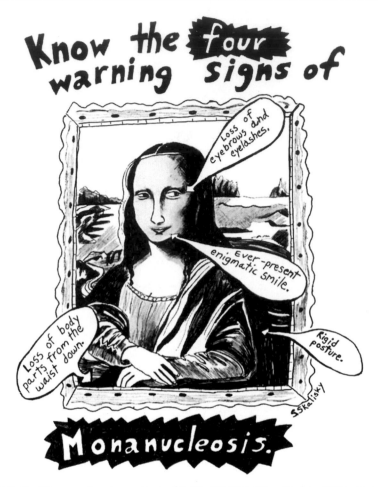

FIGURE 9. Monanucleosis cartoon, (1991). (© The New Yorker Collection 1991 Stephanie Skalisky from cartoonbank.com. All Rights Reserved)

genre promotes only narrow forms of self-doctoring, rather than dialogical forms of self-care.

The symptoms list as a genre developed in the mid-twentieth century as a means of standardizing and quantifying illnesses for the purposes of research and documentation, but its current uses have expanded far beyond this initial purpose. As an answer to a particular need among researchers to quantify symptoms and to measure their potential improvements, the symptoms list became a convenient yardstick for assessment. In the third revision of the *Diagnostic and Statistical Manual of Mental Disorders* (*DSM-III*), published in 1987, however, such lists of symptoms were imported into the descriptions of mental disorders themselves. Subsequent editions of the *DSM* have further streamlined this genre. As the official nosology of mental illness in the United States, the

DSM operates within research *and* clinical settings, so the inclusion of lists of symptoms validates the genre as a diagnostic tool in addition to its uses in the assessment of psychiatric research.[1] As the *DSM* gained professional and cultural acceptance in the last decade of the twentieth century, it became more than the arbiter of mental health and illness, it became a source that organized activities as diverse as health insurance reimbursement, legal defense claims, popular mental health speculations, and, of course, the diagnostic practices of doctors in relation to individual patients.[2] The list of depression's symptoms that might accompany an advertisement for Zoloft, for example, refers back to the *DSM*'s description, but it does so with significant modifications. The transportation of the genre from one setting to the next—from research protocol to diagnostic manual to pharmaceutical advertisement—testifies to its central role within the discourse of depression. As a tool, the symptoms list encourages practices of self-doctoring through a reconfiguration of medical expertise, and its contents gender depression and its sufferers.

A genre is more than a textual form, as the example of the symptoms list for Mononucleosis ironically points out. It is additionally a means of organizing social (inter)actions and activities: in the case of the cartoon, a list of symptoms encourages the "reading" of portraits for signs of illness. While a traditional view sees genres as sets of formal features that define texts as, for example, sonnets, detective stories, or self-help quizzes, rhetorical genre theorists see these forms as conditioning the production of texts *and* social activities within their specific contexts of use. Genres are, in Carolyn Miller's formulation, social actions.[3] Typical forms (such as the symptoms list) develop within social scenes as answers to perceived needs; they accomplish specific goals for the community members who use them. Genres and the individual texts that enact them consequently become prime artifacts in analyses of community activities.[4] Further, interactions among genres describe the broader textual landscape within which social actions succeed or fail because genres must be answered by subsequent genres—they must secure their own "uptake"—in order to take effect or trigger future responses.[5] For instance, a consultation with a doctor must be translated into the reporting codes on insurance forms in order to secure reimbursement. Similarly, the same consultation must be dictated and transcribed as notes within the patient information chart in order to constitute the patient's official medical history. In both cases, the genre of consultation must be answered by additional genres that occasion new social interactions. Within the discourse of depression, the symptoms list has been taken up in a series of consumer-based media, encouraging individuals to perform their own diagnoses and constituting new practices of self-doctoring.

Direct-to-consumer pharmaceutical advertising deploys the symptoms list as a means of promoting products. Indeed, since a 1997 FDA ruling that relaxed the restrictions on marketing pharmaceutical to consumers, doctor-patient consultations have been increasingly mediated by such texts. Yet these texts are far from objective sources of information; they produce carefully modulated messages and often target women in their appeals. In a survey of ten U.S. periodicals in 1998–1999, Steven Woloshin and colleagues note that readers of direct-to-consumer advertisements are likely to overestimate the benefits of advertised products and to expect that everyone using the products will benefit equally.[6] In another study, researchers found that women are most often the targets of this variety of pharmaceutical advertising.[7] In a telephone survey following up on these findings, approximately half of the Sacramento residents interviewed believed that such advertisements received prior approval from the FDA or another government agency (they do not).[8] Indeed, research on direct-to-consumer advertising suggests that patients increasingly rely on information they receive outside of consultations with their physicians more and more often.[9] The persuasiveness of these advertisements—measured by the number of individuals who accept illness identities and receive prescriptions to treat those identities—can be felt in expressions of anxiety about perceived overmedication.

Such anxieties surface within cartoons and jokes that appear to critique the antidepressant phenomenon. In September 1993, a *New Yorker* comic strip by Ros Chast presents "The Over-the-Counter Versions" of Peter Kramer's then-bestselling *Listening to Prozac*. "Listening to" Tylenol, Tums, and Tic Tacs, in Chast's commentary, cures a variety of troublesome symptoms: "daily aches," "inner turmoil," and "[being a] social outcast." Her cartoon echoes Kramer's claims for patients who, after taking Prozac, find themselves more vibrant, social, and confident, while implying that the same results could perhaps be achieved more economically via breath mints.[10] This humor rests on a common belief that medication has replaced resilience in the American constitution. As a result, those who use psychopharmaceuticals are judged to be weak or frivolous in their reliance on the medications. And, equally problematic, those who do not take advantage of the medications or other interventions are judged to be failing to self-doctor in culturally anticipated ways.

A second critique links depression to achievement, implying that at least some illness should not be treated. In November 1993, a *New Yorker* cartoon by Hugette Martel, speculates on what might have happened "if they had had Prozac in the nineteenth century." Karl Marx, Friedrich Nietzsche, and Edgar Allan Poe are pictured in insipidly cheerful attitudes, a prescription for Prozac having apparently erased the intellectual and cultural work each achieved in his lifetime.[11] This commentary strikes a deeper and more problematic chord that connects creativity and greatness to at least some level of depression. Medicating depression, in this view, becomes a means of stifling achievement; suffering is necessary for great thinkers, especially for great *men*. These cultural anxieties surface in the late twentieth century not simply because of the rise of popular antidepressants, but because of a public enthusiasm for writing our own prescriptions. In other words, these drugs become available for comedy when they are familiar enough to be on the tips of our tongues, which happens at least in part through the availability—in pharmaceutical advertising, online, and in informative texts—of self-diagnostic genres such as the symptoms list for depression.

Encoding Medical Expertise

Within the discourse of depression, the symptoms list in both checklist and quiz formats has become an important force in reorienting the relationships among individuals, doctors, and pharmaceuticals. To understand the symptoms list, however, we must consider how it is situated at the nexus of competing institutional, professional, and personal expectations. For standardization of research protocols and consistency of mental health care, the symptoms list serves an essential role in regulating the boundaries of depression. In its diagnostic form, the symptoms list appears in the *DSM* as a tool for medical professionals. The criteria for a Major Depressive Episode appear in summary form (figure 10) after seven pages of descriptive text that includes sections titled "Episode Features," "Associated Features and Disorders," and "Specific Culture, Age, and Gender Factors." The list itself contains cross-references to other sections of the *DSM*, and directives to users, for example, to disregard symptoms "clearly due to a general medical condition." The *DSM* symptoms list thus envisions its uptake by mental health professionals: it invokes their specialized diagnostic practices—including their knowledge of multiple disorders and their ability to judge symptoms as causing "clinically significant distress"—as prerequisites for its use. As a professional genre, then, the symptoms list constructs its users as experts who transform a series of patient experiences into symptoms of illness.

For individuals struggling with depression, however, versions of a symptoms list provide articulation and codification of their own experiences. The list invites them to envision themselves as professionals with diagnostic expertise. It becomes a signifier not only of the illness it purports to define, but also of social roles (doctors, patients), institutional structures (research funding, insurance coverage), and behavioral norms (mental health versus illness). The symptoms list is only one genre within a larger system of texts commonly used in mental health settings. Such a system can be defined by the "intertextual activity" of the texts that organize it.[12] In other words, the circulation of genres within the system—from consultation to dictation to medical history to insurance claim form—involves the repetition of terminology and standard linguistic structures from one text or genre to the next. For example, items included in the symptoms list are repeated within consultations, carrying those key

Criteria for Major Depressive Episode

A. Five (or more) of the following symptoms have been present during the same 2-week period and represent a change from previous functioning; at least one of the symptoms is either (1) depressed mood or (2) loss of interest or pleasure.

Note: Do not include symptoms that are clearly due to a general medical condition, or mood-incongruent delusions or hallucinations.

(1) depressed mood most of the day, nearly every day, as indicated by either subjective report (e.g., feels sad or empty) or observation made by others (e.g., appears tearful). **Note:** In children or adolescents, can be irritable mood.

(2) markedly diminished interest or pleasure in all, or almost all, activities most of the day, nearly every day (as indicated by either subjective account or observation made by others)

(3) significant weight loss when not dieting or weight gain (e.g., a change of more than 5% of body weight in a month), or decrease or increase in appetite nearly every day. **Note:** In children, consider failure to make expected weight gains.

(4) insomnia or hypersomnia nearly every day

(5) psychomotor agitation or retardation nearly every day (observable by others, not merely subjective feelings of restlessness or being slowed down)

(6) fatigue or loss of energy nearly every day

(7) feelings of worthlessness or excessive or inappropriate guilt (which may be delusional) nearly every day (not merely self-reproach or guilt about being sick)

(8) diminished ability to think or concentrate, or indecisiveness, nearly every day (either by subjective account or as observed by others)

(9) recurrent thoughts of death (not just fear of dying), recurrent suicidal ideation without a specific plan, or a suicide attempt or a specific plan for committing suicide

B. The symptoms do not meet the criteria for a Mixed Episode (see p. 365)

C. The symptoms cause clinically significant distress or impairment in social, occupational, or other important areas of functioning.

D. The symptoms are not due to the direct physiological effects of a substance (e.g., a drug of abuse, a medication) or a general medical condition (e.g., hypothyroidism).

E. The symptoms are not better accounted for by Bereavement, i.e., after the loss of a loved one, the symptoms persist for longer than 2 months or are characterized by marked functional impairment, morbid preoccupation with worthlessness, suicidal ideation, psychotic symptoms, or psychomotor retardation.

FIGURE 10. *DSM* criteria for a major depressive episode. American Psychiatric Association, *Diagnostic and Statistical Manual of Mental Disorders*, 4th ed., text revision (Washington, D.C.: American Psychiatric Association, 2000), 356

phrases forward into the oral genre. Similarly, doctors' awareness of required insurance forms condition the questions they ask and the information they gather from patients; their consultations anticipate the forms into which patient talk must be translated. Investigating the mental health genre system, Carol Berkenkotter and Doris Ravotas find that texts "are responsive to, refer to, index, or anticipate other texts."[13] For example, a therapist relies on her "generic expectations" as she translates a spoken patient interview into her own notes, then into an initial intake report, and finally into a health insurance claim form.[14] These translations are facilitated and to some extent motivated by the therapist's knowledge of the generic forms into which she must categorize her patients' experiences; they are a form of "generic anticipation." Such anticipation clearly structures diagnostic observations, which are additionally influenced by larger cultural discourses.

These cultural discourses, as feminist critics remind us, enter into the activities that genres organize, even into the typical content of the genres themselves. Indeed, as Hannah Lerman argues, the practice of psychodiagnosis "is inevitably linked as much—if not more—to the personality, theoretical orientation, and cultural circumstances of the therapist . . . as it is to the personality and circumstances of the patient."[15] In addition to diagnostic bias, emotional norms for women and men predispose them to different forms of "illness."[16] In the case of depression, gender differences in emotional expression are bound to skew observations of health and illness. In Western culture, for example, "the wide range of evidence of gender differences in emotional expression . . . is likely to contaminate the measurement of depression."[17] Popular understandings of femininity and masculinity shape the practice of diagnosis in part through the genre of the symptoms list, which orchestrates the psychiatric activities (such as diagnosis) within the cultural discourses (such as those regulating gendered displays of emotions) available. The use of the symptoms list by individuals repurposes the diagnostic activity toward new practices of self-doctoring.

Quizzing Ourselves Sick

Readers of women's magazines are quite familiar with the genre of the self-help quiz. These usually brief, multiple-choice tests—"Who's Your Celebrity Love Match?" and "What's Your Girlfriend Style?" and "Are You Too Picky?"[18]—are a staple of popular women's magazines and Web sites, and they offer relationship or social advice based on the respondent's final score (answers of "A" = 5 points, and so forth). In these quizzes, the "results" are often aggregated and reported in a few broad categories. For example, after completing the "Are You Too Picky?" quiz, a woman might read her evaluation under the headings: "You Deserve Better" or "Impossible to Please." Rhetorically, these social diagnostics suggest to women not only that their experiences are shared (by others in their category) but also that these experiences can be usefully understood through a short series of multiple-choice questions. For medical professionals, a similar genre—the diagnostic checklist—guides therapeutic decision making. In the *DSM*, depression becomes visible when a patient exhibits five of nine symptoms for a duration of two weeks or more (see figure 10). Rhetorically, this professional diagnostic offers a sanctioned interpretation of symptoms, legitimizes courses of treatment, and verifies eligibility for insurance reimbursement.

Read side by side, these two genres—the self-help quiz and the professional diagnostic—strongly echo each other. While there are formal differences—for example, the use of multiple-choice answers in the case of self-help quizzes, and the nominalizations of the *DSM-IV-TR* ("markedly diminished interest or pleasure")[19]—the primary difference between these genres is the contexts in which they are found. Popular women's magazines, available at local grocery and convenience stores, represent themselves as ephemeral and transitory guides to life, love, and work. The *DSM-IV-TR*, while publicly available, is certainly an example of a specialized professional text, used primarily by health care providers for the purposes of record keeping and documentation.[20] Because these contexts vary so starkly, the two genres have historically operated quite independently. In recent decades, however, the explosion of direct-to-consumer advertising has effected the merger of these two genres into a new form that works to redefine the traditional relationships among pharmaceutical companies, prospective patients, and health care providers.[21]

In the case of depression, the development of the SSRIs in the late 1980s and 1990s has coincided with the rapid increase in pharmaceutical marketing and a popular fascination with depression in the United States.[22] Most antidepressants now have dedicated Web sites, which offer versions of a depression quiz or checklist that asks the respondent to rate her (or, much less frequently, his) symptoms. Such quizzes, once taken, produce a "printable version" that the respondent is directed to take to her doctor for additional evaluation and possible treatment.[23] After answering the series of multiple-choice questions, the reader is "evaluated" by this documentation of her (or, less commonly, his) answers. Such self-diagnostic tools combine the genres of the self-help quiz (which promises casual self-assessment) and the diagnostic checklist (which provides medical evaluation), drawing on the social interactions of both. In other words, the self-diagnostic quiz at first appears as innocuous as the "Are You Too Picky?" relationship quiz. Once the reader has completed the quiz, however, the results serve as the basis for a medical encounter. By enumerating symptoms rather than experiences and by addressing a serious, medical topic, the self-diagnostic quiz appropriates the authority of the diagnostic rubric, establishing itself as a representative of the expert system of psychiatry. At the same time, however, the self-diagnostic quiz deploys a multiple-choice format and first- and second-person forms of address to create an affiliative relationship with its readers. Further, as quizzes offered by online health care information resources such as WebMD demonstrate, this genre is usually accompanied by a variety of companion genres, most notably advertisements for antidepressants. As a result, users of the quiz are situated both as experts—offered the opportunity to diagnose themselves—and as consumers of pharmaceutical products. Through the use of such genres, individuals participate in new social interactions and establish new relationships with themselves, their doctors, and various pharmaceutical companies.

The evolution of these uses can be traced in antidepressant advertisements, indicating the refinement of the genre as it is adapted to its new context and purpose. In early direct-to-consumer advertisements, the checklist is not clearly separated from the text of the advertisements; the uptake of the form itself seems to lag behind the uptake of the content. In the 1998 Prozac print advertisement (pictured in figure 2), a narrative description of depression provides readers with information they are presumed to lack.

> Depression can make you feel all alone in the world. Especially when you're around people who think depression is all in your head. Well, it's not. Depression is a real illness with real causes. It can appear suddenly, for no apparent reason. Or it can be triggered by stressful life events, like losing a job or having a chronic illness.
>
> When you're clinically depressed, one thing that can happen is the level of serotonin (a chemical in your body) may drop. *So you may have trouble sleeping. Feel unusually sad or irritable. Find it hard to concentrate. Lose your appetite. Lack energy. Or have trouble feeling pleasure.*
>
> These are some of the symptoms that can point to depression—especially if they last for more than a couple of weeks and if normal, everyday life feels like too much to handle.[24]

In this advertisement, the symptoms that "can point to depression" are listed as possible outcomes of a drop in serotonin. The symptoms themselves are mere indicators of the underlying illness; they are included for informational purposes. The Prozac advertisement goes on to claim Prozac as the "medicine doctors now prescribe most often," an implied persuasive appeal that nevertheless gives grammatical agency to doctors themselves. Similarly, the advertisement cautions that "only your doctor can decide if Prozac is right for you—or for someone you love." While clearly a promotional text, this advertisement nevertheless maintains the traditional doctor-patient social roles: the doctor will decide; the patient is to be educated.

By contrast, the 2001 print advertisement for Zoloft (pictured in figure 3) presents its case more forcefully and indicates a significant shift away from the traditional doctor-patient consultancy. In this advertisement, the symptoms are listed in bold-face type at the top of the page. Not only are they presented as a list—more akin to the professional diagnostic's format—they are also phrased as items within the consumer's knowledge (rather than the physician-expert's):

> You know when you're not feeling like yourself.
> You're tired all the time.
> You may feel sad, hopeless . . .
> and lose interest in things you once loved.
> You may feel anxious and can't even sleep.
> Your daily activities and relationships suffer.
> You know when you just don't feel right.[25]

This initial invitation to self-diagnosis is partially countermanded by a smaller-print statement that "only your doctor can diagnose depression," but the overall message to consumers in this advertisement is that *they* and not their doctors understand and interpret their own symptoms. Commanding the reader to "talk to your doctor about ZOLOFT," the advertisement explicitly enters the social interaction between doctors and patients. Instead of deferring to the doctor's judgment, the Zoloft campaign tag line—"When you know more about what's wrong, you can help make it right"—places the consumer ("you") and the pharmaceutical company (the providers of this education) into more active roles in making health care decisions. As the Zoloft advertisement has adopted the form as well as the content of the genre of the diagnostic checklist, it has assumed some of the professional authority traditionally associated with the medical tool, and yet, drawing on the popular self-help genre, it has also established a personal relationship with its readers, whose self-knowledge becomes a primary focus for the encounters.

Pharmaceutical Web sites tend to use the interactive format of the quiz rather than the static listing of symptoms, and have therefore adopted the social-interactional style of that genre most explicitly. On the Prozac Web site, the reader is directed to select one of four answers to questions such as "I am more irritable than usual" and "I still enjoy the things I used to do." When all of the answers are complete (and only then, the form will not let you submit a partial quiz), the user clicks on a "Get Your Score" button and is answered by a short message that reads: "You scored a [Number]. If you score 50 or higher, consider printing the results of your test to show your doctor." This emphasis on a "score" is highly reminiscent of popular relationship quizzes, which seek to group readers according to broad categories, but the insertion of a threshold reinforces the diagnostic authority of the quiz. A user scoring above 50 is encouraged to display the "results"—a pseudoscientific term for what amounts simply to the standardized text of each answer—for medical interpretation. Here, the quiz becomes analogous to an X-ray or the physical evidence of an illness, and the Web site becomes a referring physician, suggesting a specialized consultation. Pharmaceutical Web sites and other direct-to-consumer advertising texts have taken up both the symptoms list and the interactive quiz, as well as their accompanying social organizations. Combining the authority of the symptoms list with the affiliation and assumption of self-knowledge of the relationship quiz, the new genre of the self-diagnostic quiz participates in and helps shape the interactions between doctors and potential patients.

Individuals come to accept the illness identities resulting from their final "scores" on these quizzes, a process that happens before they enter their doctors' offices. Having completed their quizzes, individuals enter the doctor-patient consultation seeking *second* opinions. They will have already received one diagnosis through the authority of the symptoms quiz, and they will enter the doctor's office with their own "expert" conclusions sanctioned by their use of the genre. In this way, the genre itself organizes the possible social interactions among individuals and medical experts: it encourages individuals to understand themselves simultaneously as experts and as patients, and it forces doctors to offer corroborating or conflicting second opinions without the opportunity to engage in the collegial dialogue that might have accompanied traditional (human) patient referrals. In these ways, symptoms quizzes appear to streamline diagnosis, but they do so at the expense of a more dialogical engagement with the contexts, causes, and outcomes of the experiences. The genre handily reduces such experiences to symptoms in need of remediation. The characterization of these symptoms—their linguistic formulation as, for example, "I felt fearful"—becomes a second effect of the emphasis on quick diagnosis.

The Discourse of Symptoms: Gendering Depression

Whereas the forms of discourse—such as the symptoms list or quiz—help shape the social interactions possible among participants, the specific articulations— the words, images, and grammatical constructions—help define the object (in this case the depressed patient) of self-doctoring. As the symptoms list has been taken up and transformed into a self-diagnostic quiz on pharmaceutical Web sites and in print media, it has consistently marked the illness and its sufferers as feminine and isolated from their social functioning. Many of the major symptoms of depression—depressed mood, loss of pleasure, weight changes, sleep disruptions, psychomotor agitation or retardation, fatigue, feelings of worthlessness, difficulty concentrating, and thoughts of suicide—are more likely to be identified in women than in men. This apparent diagnostic bias may be partially explained by a critical reading of the language of the questionnaires and checklists that help define the illness. This language reflects the narrowing of the discourse of depression toward a gendered patient and a biological etiology.

The translations that occur in the processes of converting medical categories into quiz questions help define depression as a feminine disease. Table 6.1 compares the language of the *DSM-IV-TR* to that of three currently

TABLE 6.1

Comparison of Symptoms in Checklists for Depression

Symptom	DSM-IV-TR	Zung (Prozac.com)	PRIME-MD™ (Zoloft.com)	CES-D (NIMH)
Depressed mood	Depressed mood most of the day, nearly every day, as indicated by either subjective report (e.g., feels sad or empty) or observation made by others (e.g., appears tearful).	I feel downhearted, blue, and sad. I have crying spells or feel like it. I feel hopeful about the future. I am more irritable than usual. My life is pretty full.	Feeling down, depressed, or hopeless.	I felt that I could not shake off the blues even with help from my family. I felt depressed. I felt hopeful about the future. I was happy. I felt lonely. I had crying spells.
Loss of pleasure	Markedly diminished interest or pleasure in all, or almost all, activities most of the day, nearly every day (as indicated by either subjective account or observation made by others).	I enjoy looking at, talking to, and being with attractive men/women. I find it easy to do the things I used to. I still enjoy the things I used to do.	Little interest or pleasure in doing things.	I enjoyed life.

Weight changes	Significant weight loss when not dieting or weight gain (e.g., a change of more than 5% of body weight in a month), or decrease or increase in appetite nearly every day.	I eat as much as I used to. I notice that I am losing weight.	Poor appetite or overeating.	I did not feel like eating; my appetite was poor.
Sleep disruptions	Insomnia or hypersomnia nearly every day.	I have trouble sleeping through the night.	Trouble falling or staying asleep, or sleeping too much.	My sleep was restless.
Agitation/Retardation	Psychomotor agitation or retardation nearly every day (observable by others, not merely subjective feelings of restlessness or being slowed down).	My heart beats faster than usual. I feel restless and can't keep still.	Moving or speaking so slowly that other people notice. Or the opposite—being so fidgety or restless that you have been moving around a lot more than usual.	I talked less than usual.
Fatigue	Fatigue or loss of energy nearly every day.	I get tired for no reason.	Feeling tired or having little energy.	I felt that everything I did was an effort. I could not get "going."

(continued)

TABLE 6.1 (continued)

Symptom	DSM-IV-TR	Zung (Prozac.com)	PRIME-MD™ (Zoloft.com)	CES-D (NIMH)
Feelings of worthlessness	Feelings of worthlessness or excessive or inappropriate guilt (which may be delusional) nearly every day (not merely self-reproach or guilt about being sick).	I feel that I am useful and needed.	Feeling bad about yourself, or feeling that you are a failure or have let yourself or your family down.	I felt that I was just as good as other people. I thought my life had been a failure. I felt that people disliked me.
Difficulty concentrating	Diminished ability to think or concentrate, or indecisiveness, nearly every day (either by subjective account or as observed by others).	My mind is as clear as it used to be. I find it easy to make decisions.	Trouble concentrating on things such as reading the newspaper or watching television.	I had trouble keeping my mind on what I was doing.

Suicidal thoughts	Recurrent thoughts of death (not just fear of dying), recurrent suicidal ideation without a specific plan, or a suicide attempt or a specific plan for committing suicide.	I feel that others would be better off if I were dead.	Thinking that you would be better off dead, or wanting to hurt yourself in some way.
Other		Morning is when I feel the best. I have trouble with constipation.	I was bothered by things that usually don't bother me. I felt fearful. People were unfriendly. I felt sick.

SOURCES: Information taken from American Psychological Association, *DSM-IV-TR*, "Checklist for Major Depressive Episode" (356); "Zung Assessment Tool," Available: http://prozac.com/common_pages/quiz.jsp; "Depression Checklist," Available: http://www.zoloft.com/zoloft/zoloft.portal?_nfpb=true&_pageLabel=depr_checklist; Center for Epidemiologic Studies, National Institute of Mental Health, *CES-D*.

circulating versions of self-diagnostic tools—a quiz from Prozac.com based on the Zung Depression scale, a quiz from Zoloft.com based on PRIME-MD™, and a questionnaire (the CES-D) developed by the National Institute of Mental Health.[26] While scientific studies have confirmed that each of the underlying scales is as valid and predictive of research outcomes as the others, little rhetorical attention has been paid either to the quizzes or to the research instruments upon which they are based. Nevertheless, the three quizzes—intended for self-administration—make consequential revisions to the language of the *DSM-IV-TR*—intended for professional consultation. These articulations and translations skew toward stereotypically feminine behaviors and emotions in some cases.

For example, the *DSM-IV-TR* describes the symptom of "weight changes" as a "change of more than 5 percent of body weight in a month." In the quizzes, this is translated into "losing weight" (Zung), "poor appetite" (PRIME-MD), and "not feeling like eating" (CES-D). While these may in fact be "more accessible" criteria for patients and/or doctors, a focus on *eating* is not the same thing as a focus on rapid and drastic changes in *weight*. Further, women in our society are much more likely to notice their eating habits and to focus on "losing weight" as part of their self-maintenance.[27] In addition, only the PRIME-MD includes "overeating" in this category—the others simply ignore the possibility of weight *gain* as a symptom of depression. These quiz revisions to the *DSM* language reflect their broad attention to all forms of depression, rather than just the clinical category of Major Depressive Disorder. Indeed, some of the more colloquial language seems calibrated to identify "depression spectrum disorders" such as dysthymia, a milder but more chronic form of depression that is particularly common among women. Beyond these expansive moves, the quiz language indexes stereotypically gendered behaviors. The "Agitation/Retardation" symptom listed in the *DSM-IV-TR* as "psychomotor agitation or retardation" becomes "moving or speaking so slowly that other people notice" in the questionnaire based on the PRIME-MD and "I talked less than usual" in the CES-D. The emphasis on speaking takes up the gender stereotype that women are more verbal than men. The symptoms of depression as the questionnaires currently define them emphasize such gendered behaviors.

The language of these various quizzes focuses on excesses of emotion; depression is often conceptualized as the far end of a spectrum of grief and sadness. Yet this ambiguity—where does "normal" grief end and depression begin?—leads to difficulties when diagnostic precision is assumed to be the result of valuing responses to these questions. The translation of "depressed mood" (*DSM-IV-TR*) into "crying spells" (Zung, CES-D) may in fact make the criterion more concrete. But, it also focuses attention on a specific behavior, crying, that is more socially acceptable for women than it is for men. Further, the characterization of the episodes as "spells" evokes feminine emotional turmoil and collocates with children and immaturity, suggesting that depression sufferers are helpless and infantile. The symptoms quizzes recast the observation of a patient's "tearful" appearance in the *DSM-IV-TR* as an uncontrollable storm, performing uptakes of emotional commonplaces that help to feminize the illness and its sufferers.

Beyond the emphasis on feelings, the symptoms quizzes also draw out social and family relationships as being significant factors in the diagnosis of depression. The *DSM-IV-TR* criteria note in several places that symptoms may be self-reported or observed by others, but no mentions of peers or family are made in the official document. By contrast, all three of the questionnaires refer to social groups and families. The Zung quiz refers to the enjoyment of "looking at, talking to, and being with attractive men/women." This item—one of the "reverse" questions in the quiz that helps ensure readers are carefully attending to each question—clearly implies that one should enjoy these social activities. The PRIME-MD asks about "feeling that you . . . have let yourself or your family down," introducing the family unit into the diagnostic apparatus. Similarly, the CES-D asks about "the blues," which cannot be shaken "even with the help from my family," and also about feelings that "people disliked me." Each of these quiz items helps reinforce the "healthiness" of social relationships, and marks the failures of such relationships as potential symptoms of illness. Significantly, the transformation of the impersonal diagnostic criteria of the *DSM-IV-TR* into first- and second-person statements reinforces the personal responsibility of the individual, while it simultaneously removes the possibility of peer and family reporting of symptoms. The individual is rhetorically isolated even as she is asked to rate her own social functioning.

The texts used to diagnose and identify depression regulate not only what counts as illness but also what roles we expect of patients and health care providers in relation to it. When individuals invoke "the list" of symptoms for depression as a single discursive unit, as they do in the interviews described below, they begin the process of abstracting their experiences from the narrative fabric of their lives. Giving up the particularities of their individual encounters with these symptoms, their uses of the phrase "the list" leave unchallenged the ideological implications of the definition as it is constructed within the genre. Further, these utterances vest the individuals with responsibility for managing their new medical conditions, usually through pharmaceutical interventions.

Defining the Self in Women's Talk about Depression

To accept the label *depressed* is to take up the implied and explicit definitions of that illness identity. To make use of the genre of the symptoms list is to accept crucial elements of its authority and its social explanatory powers. Laurie, a clinical psychologist, describes her strategies for recruiting women for her research studies on depression, saying: "The one time we ever advertised for depressed women, we got no one. The minute we started putting the symptoms out, we got tons of people coming in. I think it was some of that, that stigma stuff where they didn't, you know, (A) no one had been diagnosed, and then (B) they didn't want to come in for a study on depression. But if you said, 'Are you feeling sad? Are you feeling alone? Are you feeling blue? Is it hard to get up in the mornings?' it was like, 'That's me.'" Rather than advertising for "depressed women," Laurie reports that she and her clinical staff have better luck when they use the terminology of a symptoms quiz. Laurie speculates that this is in part due to the stigma still associated with the term *depressed*. More telling, however, is the fact that the women who do respond to the questions Laurie substitutes for the label—Are you feeling sad? Are you feeling alone?— appear to recognize not just their experiences but also their *selves* in the constellation of symptoms.

This recognition of self within a series of symptoms of depression is a practice that receives careful nurturing among texts written for the youngest of readers. *The Feelings Book*, a 2002 publication in the popular American Girl™ series, encourages, in the words of its subtitle, "the care and keeping of your emotions." Within this book, a variety of record-keeping activities are encouraged as means of coping with one's feelings. The genre conventions of diagnostic quizzes for depression are followed in the text's "Mood-o-Meters" (figure 11). Asking readers—typically aged eight to eleven years old—to rate the severity of their emotions in response to specific scenarios, the "temperature" of each emotion is given verbal expression. For example, sadness at leaving home for the entire summer is codified along the scale from "I'll miss my room at home" to "I'd call this 'super-sob sad.'" This gamelike record keeping is preparatory for the more serious self-monitoring required to be assured of mental health. Such charting of moods draws on the psychiatric tradition at least as far back as the early twentieth century, when Emil Kraepelin published his work on manic depression. In the 2003 *Judy Moody Mood Journal*, a "temperamental third-grade girl" helps young readers learn to chart their own feelings. Such texts, in Emily Martin's analysis, teach children "to take individual responsibility for managing [their interior] states. The record keeping of moods thus extends from children whose moods cause problems at school or home to (potentially) all children."[28] A new generation of consumers is thus being trained to use the genres that will eventually require their own self-doctoring.

At another point in *The Feelings Book*, readers are provided with a list of the symptoms of depression and directed to show their results—the number of items that apply to them—to an adult, who may refer the child (and her results) directly to a doctor. This chain of events depicts self-monitoring as the first step in a process whereby the individual submits to medical care. While in some cases this submission is necessary and beneficial, the genre and the social organization it produces bypass a number of social interactions that might also be appropriate interventions. The book encourages young girls to "unpack" their emotions of jealousy, fear, and anger at their friends, but sadness—the precursor to depression—is treated more seriously as a potentially medical condition. Textual representations such as the "Mood-O-Meter" which makes a game of a potentially consequential interaction and the symptoms quiz train girls and women to recognize them*selves* and not just their experiences in the symptoms of depression. As a result, they become perfect consumers of the antidepressant medications, which often sponsor the texts that offer such familiar self-assessments.

Beyond this self-recognition, the list of symptoms as a whole has become a convenient shorthand for referring to a group of feelings and experiences. In their conversations about depression and mental health more generally, the women I spoke with refer to the symptoms of depression as established facts and as a coherent unit: "the list." The women take up the genre of the symptoms list as a single (and stable) entity, rather than interrogating or even enumerating its contents. By doing so, they accept the contours of the illness and the gendered identities codified in the genre. Such a reduction of suffering (an experiential entity) to mere symptoms (diagnostic entities) empties suffering of its social and moral significance.[29] The shorthand of symptoms masks the complexities of lived experiences and ignores the value of suffering to promote ethical social behaviors. "The list" consequently represents a challenge to a rhetorical self-definition; without delineating the specific symptoms, the women appear to accept and recirculate the gendered construction of depression itself.

The women's evocations of the symptoms list demonstrate this emptying or forgetting of the narrative trajectory of their illness experiences. The list holds power as a synecdoche for a larger expert system of diagnosis and treatment. It operates at the level of a dead metaphor, being used by the women as a self-evident and transparent frame that verifies their illness identities. In fact, the symptoms list at times eclipses the expertise of mental health professionals themselves. Not only do the women identify the list of symptoms as a single discursive unit, but they also set the authority of this list against and above the authority of health care professionals. Claire, a graduate student in the humanities, relates her recent visit to the campus health center by saying, "I was in last month. I went to Campus Health and talked to a woman in there. And she asked me questions, and I told her my symptoms, which are all on the list. And she didn't, you know, say 'you're depressed.' She said it sounded that way, and [she] recommended counseling and medication." In Claire's narrative, an important feature is the erasure of her individual symptoms in favor of the more generalized "list." She reports that the campus health professional asked

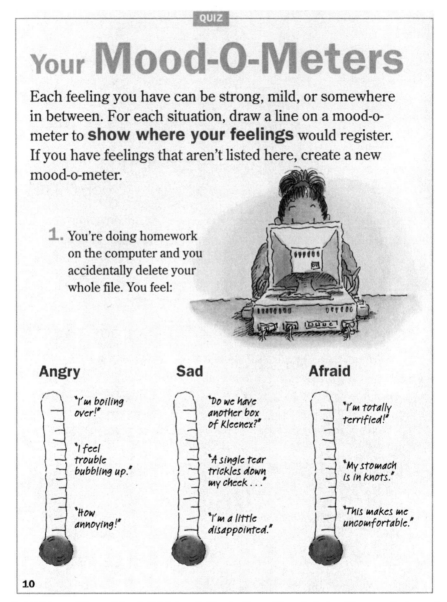

FIGURE 11. "Your Mood-O-Meters" illustration. (Reprinted with permission of American Girl Publishing from *The Feelings Book* © copyright 2000 by American Girl, LLC)

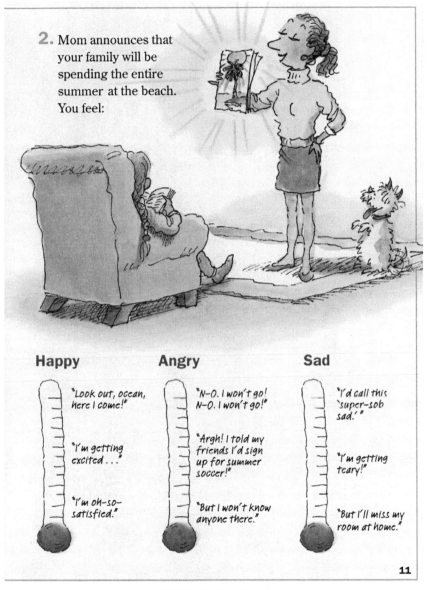

2. Mom announces that your family will be spending the entire summer at the beach. You feel:

Happy	Angry	Sad
"Look out, ocean, here I come!"	"N–O. I won't go! N–O. I won't go!"	"I'd call this 'super-sob sad.'"
"I'm getting excited..."	"Argh! I told my friends I'd sign up for summer soccer!"	"I'm getting teary!"
"I'm oh-so-satisfied."	"But I won't know anyone there."	"But I'll miss my room at home."

11

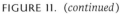

FIGURE 11. (*continued*)

her questions to which she responded with her symptoms, "which were all on the list." Here, Claire assumes a common knowledge of a stable (and complete) list of symptoms of depression. By bracketing her own experience in this way, she accepts the diagnosis offered by the symptoms list itself; she translates her particular experiences into a set of medically visible symptoms. Further, she casts doubt on the reliability of the health center professional (whom she calls "a woman in there") because she does not immediately recognize Claire's symptoms as fulfilling the checklist for depression. Instead, Claire reports that the health care provider "didn't . . . say 'you're depressed.'" Thus, the symptoms list appears to carry more diagnostic certainty for Claire than the health care provider's judgment. Claire's interaction with the campus health center is structured by her use of the symptoms list as an interpretative and self-diagnostic tool. The health care provider seems to agree with the list's diagnosis and recommends appropriate treatment, but Claire's representation of this encounter displays her confidence in the list of symptoms and foregrounds her own rhetorical presentation and self-definition (via "the list") as occurring prior to the health care encounter.

Claire repeats the elision of individual symptoms of depression again a few minutes later in our conversation, when she describes a television commercial for a research study that she has recently seen:

KE: What other commercials have you seen? Have you seen any other ads?

CLAIRE: Well, I've seen the 292–CARE research study where you can be a volunteer.

KE: What's the commercial like? What do you remember about it?

CLAIRE: It just tells you the symptoms: do you blah blah blah. If so, you may be eligible for this, um, depression study.

KE: And, did you identify with it?

CLAIRE: Mmm hmm.

Claire reports the content of the commercial, but this time she replaces the details of the symptoms of depression with "blah blah blah." She again relies on her interlocutors' shared knowledge of the symptoms rather than elaborating on them as individual entities. Treating the symptoms in this way, Claire adopts an uncritical stance toward them: they form part of a common stock of facts, rather than a culturally determined set of guidelines. Further, her identification with the commercial also signals her acceptance of the illness identity offered by the list of symptoms: she believes she is depressed, and she believes this because her symptoms match a uniform list that represents a single diagnosis. Yet the list itself may in fact hide additional important symptoms and also social and environmental contexts that are relevant to health and illness experiences.[30] Symptoms of illness are based in discrete individual experiences, but when they are grouped together as an abstract entity—"the list"—they lose even this specificity. Further, the abstraction of each symptom renders unnecessary the possible explanations for it: "feelings of hopelessness," described as a single symptom, are divorced from their possible social causes (e.g., the loss of a job or a loved one, or the experience of racial or economic inequality). The value of the symptoms list is its ability to help individuals such as Claire recognize their health care needs; the danger of this list appears in its ability to seem complete and to keep individuals from recognizing other health care options.

As part of the recruiting procedures for the interviews, I asked the women who volunteered to talk with me to complete the CES-D depression questionnaire. This allowed me to select individuals who indicated a moderate but not clinical level of symptoms. As we talked together, I asked the women to discuss the experience of interacting with that symptoms questionnaire. I asked about their reactions to the form they completed:

KE: When you filled out the screening materials for this study, that symptoms questionnaire? Tell me a little bit about your reaction to that. It was the check boxes, "I've felt this way: Rarely, Sometimes"=

STEPH: =I wanted to check between the boxes. Like okay, last week this happened, oh that's not quite the same as 3 or 4, it was kind of 2 and 3. I probably tried, but I- I've kind of forced them into categories for simplicity's sake. . . .

MEI: Well, I just, I guess it was just nice. I mean if you asked me to write it out, I might not have written all the symptoms. But then checking the box was like: yeah, yeah, I do have that [laughs] and like=

STEPH: =yes, that, oh yeah, that on occasion too=

MEI: =yeah

STEPH: It was kind of a convenient compartmentalizing experience. Oh, yes, this is what this is. Oh, wow, other people feel—this is so validating.

MEI: [Laughs] Yeah.

Initially, Stephanie expresses her frustration with the genre—she "wanted to check between the boxes" rather than conforming to the genre's four categories (less than 1 day, 1–2 days, 3–4 days, 5–7 days). But as the conversation continues, Mei reports that the experience of filling in the survey helps her clarify her experiences as part of the illness, depression. The women in this study were chosen specifically because they did *not* score highly enough on the CES-D index to be considered clinically depressed, so it is notable that the form itself still works to validate Mei's personal sense that she is, in fact, depressed. Mei admits that she would not necessarily be able to write down all of her symptoms, but that she recognizes them when she sees them in the CES-D. This recognition suggests that the genre itself does both rhetorical and diagnostic work for the individuals who use it. The women use the form as a means of articulating something they feel but for which they do not have terminology, but, in the process, they also consent to the form's diagnostic imperative. After her initial expressions of frustration, Stephanie describes the form as "convenient" and "validating." The genre indicates to her that others feel as she does; the authority of the form works to help her define her own experiences.

These women reveal themselves to be active participants in their own discursive construction as depressed (or not depressed) individuals. Their use of the symptoms list as a single discursive unit suggests that this genre has, indeed, become a significant determiner of illness identity. To qualify for diagnosis, one must have symptoms "on the list" and must represent oneself through that rhetorical lens in order to be recognized. More significantly, the women make use of the genre of the symptoms list to create personally meaningful identities. Stephanie and Mei find the genre a useful tool for categorizing and explaining their experiences. These self-constructed meanings are not, however, uncomplicated or free from rhetorical valences. As they accept the validity and stability of the genre's definition of depression, the women adopt institutionally recognizable language that genders their identities and conditions a narrow range of possible (pharmaceutical) interventions into their experiences.

The growth of the self-diagnostic quiz as both a marketing vehicle and an educational tool raises important questions for medical rhetoricians and for individuals who choose to make use of it. The women who spoke with me confirm the importance of this new genre in the construction and comprehension of depression as an illness, but they also suggest that it imparts certainty and medical authority that the individual texts often deny (as seen in the legal disclaimers and notices that accompany them). How, then, does a symptoms quiz take up the social functions—primarily of diagnosis and prescription—that have traditionally been performed only by physicians? The answer, in part, lies in the effectiveness of pharmaceutical campaigns that deploy the new hybrid tool, the self-diagnostic quiz, to exploit a new rhetorical position within the health care system. Individual readers of such advertising (and educational) materials similarly make use of the new genre as a part of their own self-definition. The symptoms quiz becomes an important site for rhetorical investigation, directing our gaze toward the ongoing reconfiguration of health care in the United States.

What comes to be recognized as illness (rather than, for example, as "normal" sadness or grief) is a construction of repeated textual performances within recognized diagnostic genres.[31] Each text, from definition to patient rehearsal of symptoms, reinforces the stability of that construction. As individuals interact with the texts and genres, they take up the social roles available to them, the contours of the illness itself, and, eventually, they may also take up the material (pharmaceutical) responses to depression. Such ideological management of individuals' experiences encourages new patient activities, including transforming narrative events into medical symptoms and demanding pharmaceutical interventions. Nevertheless, such activities are also occasions for the construction of personally meaningful self-representations and recognitions, as they seem to be for Mei and Stephanie.

As they make use of the symptoms list, these women nevertheless reorient themselves toward the biomedical institutions. Stephanie's initial desire to "check between the boxes" is rapidly transformed into an acceptance of the genre's authority. Yet in her initial response I see room for practices beyond the narrow, pharmaceutical desires of self-doctoring; I see the opportunity to develop a rhetorical care of the self that does not break free from the discourse of depression, but rather consciously uses it to achieve personally meaningful ends. It is only a brief vision, though, and one that is too quickly overridden by her peers' commentary, which Stephanie takes on and amplifies in her subsequent responses. The dismissive query of the *New Yorker* cartoon in figure 1— "How's the self-diagnosis going?"—highlights the dangers of uncritically adopting the genres offered as efficiencies in the health care system. Too often, such tools elide the lived realities and constructed experiences of individuals. The power vested in genres, especially when those genres participate in foundational texts such as the *DSM*, has been harnessed most effectively within the strategies of direct-to-consumer marketing. As an important feature within the discourse of depression, the genre of the self-diagnostic symptoms quiz reveals patterns of self-doctoring as well as potential occasions for a rhetorical care of the self.

Conclusion

Toward a Rhetorical Care of the Self

As a rhetorical analysis of the symptoms quiz for depression shows, what often passes for "care" in the discourse of depression is, in fact, self-doctoring. Texts that appear to promote personal autonomy and dialogue turn out to have gendered identities embedded within them. As individuals take such texts for granted, they cease to question the authority or validity of their uses of them; like the women who spoke with me, they begin to feel reassured by the familiarity of the selves they encounter through the stories and genres that help construct depression as a common mental illness. The discourse of depression constantly evolves, and it reflects the interests of the powerful social and bio-medical institutions that generate many of the now familiar texts. Strategies that may have begun as attempts to promote self-care (for example, the government informational brochures produced by NIMH) are likely to be co-opted and redirected toward these institutions' narrow biomedical disease models. Nevertheless, a critical reading of texts about depression might help individuals live under health and illness descriptions with more consciousness and therefore more flexibility in their personal responses.

Such rhetorical self-care originates in a fundamental curiosity about the self and its relationship with the social and physical worlds. It works within circulating discourses to seek opportunities for tactical responses to those discourses, responses that bring personally meaningful experiences to individuals. It cannot operate outside of the coercive discourses that instill the self-doctoring drive, so it must remain dynamic in order to make tactical use of opportunities as they appear. Because the strategies that compel individuals to doctor themselves are deployed by powerful institutions such as pharmaceutical companies, counterstrategies that create opportunities for self-care must also be fostered among powerful social entities (which may, perhaps, even include those same pharmaceutical companies). Such sites include educational and medical institutions, which can nurture the habits of critical reading and dialogic engagement with the discourses of health and illness. Such engagement promises to bridge the previously uncrossable divides between literary analysis and clinical practice, between subjective description and objective classification, and between patient and doctor. This humanistic impulse is particularly necessary in an era of increased abstractions away from the self, an era exemplified by faith in biology, genetics, and brain chemistry, rather than social exchange and inquiry.

Rediscovering the Narratives in Medicine

Within the discourse of depression, a loss of storytelling represents a loss of self-care. For author and psychologist Lauren Slater, faith in pure science at the expense of human interaction characterizes contemporary psychopharmacology. She describes this branch of treatment as the one place "where there is no need for intimacy; neither knives nor stories are an essential part of its practice. And in its understandable glee that it might finally move psychiatry into a position as respectable as surgery, it risks forgetting, or maybe never learning, what even many a surgeon knows: that you must smooth the skin, that you must stop by the bedside in your blue scrub suit, that language is the kiss of life."[1] For Slater, the physical intimacy of language brings humanity to medicine; it connects doctors with patients and patients with their own storied lives. Knowing that there is a variety of cultural narratives about Prozac, Slater begins her memoir by refuting their easy solutions that tell only the master narrative of the triumph of biomedicine: "No. For me the story of Prozac lies . . . in a place my doctor was not taught to get to—the difficulty and compromise of cure, the grief and light of illness passing, the fear as the walls of the hospital wash away and you have before you this—this strange planet, pressing in."[2] Her story is thus one of interpretation rather than one of restitution; it is also an individual, precise story of selfhood.

Slater writes of learning how to read "this strange planet" (i.e., the landscape of health) through the focalization of Prozac; she writes of her alienation from the Prozac Doctor, who becomes a caricature of biomedicine. It is the alienation of having been stripped of her own narrative. She writes that "[the Prozac Doctor] had all the right gestures. His knowledge was impeccable. He made eye contact with the subject, meaning me. But still, there was something about the way the Prozac Doctor looked at me, and the very technical way he spoke to me, that made me feel he was viewing me generally—swf, long psych history, five hospitalizations for depression and anxiety-related problems, poor medication response in past, now referred as outpatient for sudden OCD—as opposed to me, viewing me, in my specific skin."[3] The Prozac Doctor's failure to see Slater as an individual, and his incomprehension of the narratives that surround his interactions with her, construct her as nothing more than a generalization, a case. Even as he proffers his response—a pill in place of a conversational or narrative turn—he holds "himself so politely, angled away from contact."[4] Indeed, it is *contact*, but also a specific kind of *narrative* contact, that Slater misses in her interactions with biomedical institutions. Her memoir serves as an attempt to reestablish connections with herself and the world.

Opening such communicative passages between isolated individuals, Rita Charon's *Narrative Medicine* builds relationships between physicians and patients. Her program at the College of Physicians and Surgeons at Columbia University responds to a demand, like Slater's, for contact through the exchange of stories. Bridging two isolated disciplinary spaces, narrative medicine allows insight to pass between the arts and the sciences. According to Charon, "medicine, nursing, social work, and other health care professions need proven means to singularize the care of patients, to recognize professionals' ethical and personal duties toward the sick, and to bring about healing relationships with patients, among practitioners, and with the public."[5] Here, narrative can "singularize the care of patients" by restoring their individuality and perhaps their agency—through the telling of their own stories—to medical interactions. Narrative can, in other words, serve as a powerful tool for promoting the rhetorical care of the self. Charon also suggests that "literary studies and narrative theory . . . seek practical ways to transfer their conceptual knowledge into palpable influence in the world, and a connection with health care can do that."[6] A connection to the "practical" within health care interactions thus explains for literary study the physical effects of stories, which have been ignored in more aesthetic traditions. Charon contends that "by telling stories to ourselves and others . . . we grow slowly not only *to know* who we are but also *to become* who we are."[7] The first is a matter of reading comprehension, the second of transformation. Comprehension requires what Charon calls "narrative competence," which includes "the skills needed to listen to narratives of illness, to understand what they mean, to attain rich and accurate interpretations of these stories, and to grasp the plight of patients in all their complexity."[8] Beyond the clinical and scientific skills of medicine, such narrative competence encourages health care professionals to attend to patients as individuals and as protagonists in their own lives. Reciprocally, narrative competence might be extended to patients, who stand to benefit from the similar humanizing of their health care providers.

Certainly a narrative medicine can help patients and physicians know each other in more meaningful ways, but the second outcome of narrative medicine—the transformation of selves—is less easily accounted for by the platitudes of personalized health care that result from attending to these stories. In the end, narratives do seem to help make sense of who we are and how our experiences may be integrated into our lives. They serve as connective tissue between isolated individuals, and they cross professional, disciplinary, and social divides. But, to the extent that narratives serve as persuasive models through which individuals construct their own identities, a *rhetorical* competence must complement Charon's version of narrative competence. In other words, stories must be understood not simply as communicative vehicles but also as powerful shapers of the available identities within discursive frames such as the discourse of depression.[9]

Encouraging physicians to attend to the stories of their patients, narrative medicine proponents argue, provides better and more ethical health care. Charon suggests physicians develop their narrative competence through three stages of engagement: attention, representation, and affiliation. First, "Attention connotes the emptying of self so as to become an instrument for receiving the meaning of another."[10] This practice encourages physicians to listen carefully and meaningfully to their patients, rather than drawing on their own experiences and expertise (steps that presumably come after the patient's story is heard in full). The narrative "representation" of patients' stories, a second stage of engagement, serves as a necessary corollary to attention because it allows the physician to understand the experiences of the patient. The final step toward achieving narrative competence is the "affiliation" that results from the reciprocal practices of attention and representation. For Charon, the practice of narrativizing her patients' experiences enables her to "become invested in the patient's singular situation."[11] She comes to attend to the *expression* of their stories, to the unique details that affect their care. Together the practices of attention, representation, and affiliation shape a more ethical, because more personal and situated, medical care.

Charon's three-part model encourages the alignment of physician and patient, but it might be equally well applied to the alignment between individual and the wider discourse of depression. Attending to the gendered illness identities available within the definitions, metaphors, stories, and genres of the discourse of depression, individuals learn to represent *themselves* within those structures. Having done so, they naturally *affiliate* with the solutions—primarily psychopharmaceutical—offered within the discourse. In this way, the ethical achievement of narrative medicine might lead individuals to *more* rather than *fewer* self-doctoring practices. What is missing for individuals confronting the discourse of depression is a *rhetorical* competence that adds to the narrative competence Charon describes for physicians. Individuals in their daily lives are confronted not with an opportunity tell their stories—as in the controlled encounter within the doctor's office—but with the compulsion to author themselves on an ongoing basis. Such self-construction certainly attends to stories, but it also makes use of the already circulating rhetorical structures and ideologies. Therefore, individuals must develop more complex tactics that include, but go beyond, narrative competence.

The mental health professionals who spoke with me seem to recognize this need when they begin to discuss the individuality of each depression. As they work with patients to recognize the illness, Betty, Ellen, and Joan construct a powerfully contingent definition of depression:

BETTY: Oh, the first thing they tell me, a lot of them, is that they're feeling depressed. That's the first thing they tell me.

KE: Just straight out: "I'm feeling depressed"?

BETTY: Mmm hmmm. "I'm depressed." And then it takes about an hour to figure out what's really going on [laughs]. That's the entry they have to get into my office, but then it takes about an hour to figure out what else is going on. They may not be depressed; it may be just the way to get in.

ELLEN: Me too. . . . typically the first thing they say is, "I'm depressed." And, and then it does take an hour to figure out what that really means to them. And to tease out whether they're something else in addition to being depressed.

JOAN: I think that really speaks to this whole idea that we keep coming back to: how sort of nonuniform it [i.e., depression] is.

OTHERS: Mmm hmm.

This conversation between Betty and Ellen explains why their initial consultations may bewilder some of their patients. Their patients arrive having already determined for themselves that they are depressed, even if this determination may not be medically accurate. Instead of immediately agreeing with these self-diagnoses, both Betty and Ellen take an hour to "figure out what's really going on" in the individual patient's life story. Elsewhere in our conversation, Ellen describes her own rhetorical strategy: she asks patients how they know they are *becoming depressed* as a means of encouraging them to unpack their initial declarations. Such questions—the heart, I presume, of the time she and Betty take with patients—aim at developing a rhetorical competence in individuals. If individuals can come to understand the complexities of their "simple" statements—such as "I'm depressed"—they might be able to engage in a rhetorical self-care that *reads* the self alongside its many discursive representations (pharmaceutical, gendered, isolated, socially responsible) as opposed to simply affiliating the self with one (or more) of those representations.

Just such an impulse to foster critical reading and reflection motivates rhetorical engagements with discourses of health and illness. For example, a better *understanding* of the language system from which medical records derive—based in the data collection measures of the *DSM-III*—could be an empowering form of knowledge for patients and physicians. As many scholarly disciplines acknowledge, information is available for multiple interpretations, depending on its context, audience, and purpose. Much of the information produced about depression—for example, the NIMH brochures and news stories—tends to recirculate the linguistic structures and biomedical strategies that encourage self-doctoring, but such information might still serve as the basis for counterstrategies aimed at producing a rhetorical care of the self. Government informational campaigns and those of private interest groups offer educational interventions to help individuals recognize the signs and symptoms of depression. Such materials can be used to open rather than close conversations, but this requires that the texts circulate *in dialogue* with others, and that the texts are not substituted for the contact among social networks that often erodes during depression. The *Blues Buster* newsletter—which was discontinued in 2004—offered another counterstrategy to the circulating discourse of depression, providing a vehicle for distributing new information about research on depression. Online support groups and discussion boards likewise offer a means of disseminating knowledge. But each of these strategies requires a rhetorical orientation toward the information presented. Information by itself is not the answer; it must be accompanied by a series of critical reading strategies that place the information in the context of the audience for whom it was produced and in which it appears. Therefore, as a concluding thought experiment, I propose a curriculum for an interdisciplinary course within the medical humanities that might begin to foster such critiques and to offer students the opportunities they need to make tactical choices that promote self-care.

Reading the Discourse of Depression: An Interdisciplinary Seminar

The mental health crisis on U.S. college campuses has been widely proclaimed. In 2004, *Newsweek* reported that a "survey by the American College Health Association, more than 40 percent of students reported feeling 'so depressed, it was difficult to function' at least once during the year; 30 percent said they were suffering from an anxiety disorder or depression. . . . In January [2004] the *Crimson*, Harvard's student newspaper, published a widely discussed five-part series concluding that 'an overwhelming majority' of Harvard undergraduates experience mental-health problems. The series further stated that the university's shortcomings in helping students were causing 'a pervasive mental-health crisis.'"[12] In response to this crisis, my own university has increased its use of online quasi-diagnostic tools for illnesses such as depression. On the University Counseling Services Web site, students can find and take a variety of "mental health screenings" and participate in "Healthy Choice Clinics," which offer drop-in opportunities for students "to discuss concerns they have about sleep, substance abuse and stress or anxiety." In addition to these clinics, University Counseling Services sponsors a number of support groups, including

"Managing Stress through Meditation," "Self-Management and Recovery Training" (an alternative to twelve-step programs), and "Coping with Grief and Loss." Although there is no group specifically for depressed students, the online screening tools offer symptoms quizzes for depression, bipolar disorder, generalized anxiety disorder, and posttraumatic stress disorder. These tools appear to be the first interaction many students on my campus might have with the Counseling Services office.

On Facebook, a popular social networking site—which my students report consulting and updating many times a day—a simple search for the term "depression," returns over five hundred "groups." For example, the "Depression and Suicide Awareness Campaign—In Memory of Andrei Lehman," which is based in Ohio, maintains a page that chronicles the development of a depression-awareness campaign by Lehman's father. The page includes a narrative of Lehman's death and additional utilities such as a discussion board, announcements, photos, and a public "wall" on which Lehman's friends have posted comments and others have suggested additional resources and groups within Facebook. As of April 2009, the group included 429 members. Another group, "Four guys, one destination, one mission: suicide prevention," has nearly 260,000 members following the cycling tour of four young men on a mission to promote awareness of suicide prevention strategies. Virtual communities—such as those on Facebook—offer new rhetorical scenes in which depression information circulates. But, despite much media attention directed toward social networking, there have been no sustained analyses of the rhetoric of such support group sites. Facebook and University Counseling Services are locations that students might analyze in order to develop the critical reading strategies characteristic of a rhetorical care of the self.

Reading such sites is, however, only a monological activity unless those readings are placed in dialogue with other texts, contexts, and audiences. Therefore, I propose using educational institutions themselves to encourage tactical responses to powerful discourses of health and illness. One such intervention might be an interdisciplinary seminar in which students participate in experiential learning activities, which require them to spend at least three hours per week in a professional health care setting. My university sits directly between the campuses of two major research hospitals; the city Free Medical Clinic is within walking distance of campus; and the University Counseling Services office provides another venue for such student interaction. In each health care setting, students might gather texts that define health and illness and, eventually, choose one to work with and revise throughout the semester. Rewriting the text in a variety of modes and for a variety of audiences will help students come to understand the complexity of the rhetorical construction of health and illness. The learning outcomes of such a seminar include developing students' abilities to contextualize written materials within their historical,

professional, and social settings; to read and write within a range of disciplinary conventions; to perform critical rhetorical analyses on health care documents; and to present the results of the semester's inquiry back to the health
care institutions at which they are volunteering. This basic course structure
might be applied to a variety of topical seminars, but the course I am envisioning here engages explicitly with the discourse of depression.

In a fifteen-week semester, students might attend to depression from five
disciplinary standpoints—historical, literary, sociological, biological, and
rhetorical—producing appropriate texts that contribute to the final project for
the course: a substantial revision of a text that their service site uses to define,
illustrate, or respond to depression. The students' revisions account not merely
for new content or for the needs of another audience, but also for a new social
or rhetorical medium (e.g., by producing a Web page, a video, a graphical flyer
for individuals who are not literate, or a similar radical re-visioning of the text).
As they prepare for these complex revisions—the primary project for their fifth
and final disciplinary unit—students work through materials from other modes
of inquiry. For example, in a unit on the history of depression, students might
read from Jennifer Radden's *Nature of Melancholy* and assemble a documentary
archive from their health care sites and from other available collections. In a
unit on literature and depression, students could read Elizabeth Wurtzel's
Prozac Nation and write their own personal illness narrative. In a unit on the
sociology of depression, they would read David Karp's *Speaking of Sadness* and
interview users about the experience of reading mental health brochures
(a form of "usability testing" that will enable students to gather reactions to
text design). Finally, in a unit on the biology of depression, students should
attend to research summarized in the Public Library of Science and produce an
annotated bibliography of recent research studies.

In the summative unit of the seminar—a unit on rhetorical approaches to
depression—students would reread the texts for the semester through the lens
of rhetorical analysis, guided by Richard Gwyn's *Communicating Health and
Illness*. These rereadings aim at rewriting the texts that students have chosen
from their service sites. This activity encourages students to reflect on both the
original and their revised texts, and it also asks them to prepare a critical reflection essay that justifies the choices made in their processes of revision. At the
end of the seminar, students will have engaged with multiple frameworks for
depression; they will have produced a text that makes tactical use of the opportunities afforded by the dialogue between frameworks. This brief description
only scratches the surface of the possibilities for students and teachers in
college classrooms. Nevertheless, it suggests a means of supporting and promoting tactical responses to powerful and coercive discourses of health and
illness. Educational institutions have the resources and cultural capital to
engage critically with such discourses, but they rarely marshal their forces in

the collaborative, interdisciplinary way I am envisioning here. The specialization of U.S. higher education works against the rich possibilities for sharing knowledge and opening dialogue across disciplinary boundaries. It is my hope that in the process of developing interdisciplinary seminars in the rhetoric of health care, faculty might serve as a model for their students, who, when they graduate, will have to navigate the discursive terrain without the structure of a course syllabus to direct their attention to intersecting interests and motivations.

THE DISCOURSE OF DEPRESSION—indeed all health discourses—gives shape and form to the illness identities that can be taken on by individuals. At the turn of the twenty-first century, those identities have been constructed largely around the needs of a growing pharmaceutical industry. They have additionally been gendered in ways that predispose women to suspect their emotional experiences and men to disregard theirs. The resulting "biochemical self" engages in practices of self-doctoring that comply with these gendered identities and that facilitate the submission of the self to pharmaceutical intervention. At times, such self-doctoring is both necessary and expedient. Individuals must—within the social and rhetorical contexts in which they live—choose the responses that most closely align with their perceived needs. When self-doctoring is unreflective, however, when individuals come to assume that neurotransmitter balances can be measured and regulated precisely (as opposed to approximately), or when they simply assume a woman's response to grief will be clinical depression, they must be challenged to perform a more critical and rhetorical care of the self. The discursive impulse toward narrow practices of self-doctoring is multifaceted and deeply embedded in all of the ways that depression is defined, so to encourage a rhetorical self-care requires a constant reevaluation of the definitions, metaphors, stories, genres, and other rhetorical structures that define mental health and illness. Fostering a rhetorical care of the self does not imply an antipsychiatry stance, nor does it set itself against traditional biomedicine, or align itself with holistic healing. Rather, it implies an orientation toward *all* of those institutions, one that is carefully critical and open to dialogue. Helping individuals read and live rhetorically may, in the end, be our only option within the contemporary discursive contexts of health and illness; it may also be good medicine.

NOTES

INTRODUCTION: DEPRESSION AND GENDER
IN THE AGE OF SELF-CARE

1. Andrew Solomon, *The Noonday Demon: An Atlas of Depression* (New York: Scribner, 2001), 300 (emphasis added).

2. The gender of this "patient" is important: as Allan Horwitz comments, a "culture of mental health . . . is now the everyday reality of daytime talk shows, television series, popular magazines for girls and women (and sometimes men), and virtually all advice columnists" (*Creating Mental Illness* [Chicago: University of Chicago Press, 2002], 4). This relatively recent and gendered culture of mental health, Horwitz points out, is particularly evident in media directed at girls and women. In addition, women are more likely to search for health information online. According to the Health on the Net Foundation, 72 percent of patients in the United States who responded to a recent Internet usage survey were women.

3. Amy Harmon, "Young, Assured and Playing Pharmacists to Friends," *New York Times*, November 16, 2005.

4. Throughout this book, I will be using brand names for a variety of antidepressant medications. Trademarks for each of these brand names are registered by the manufacturers. For convenience, I list the manufacturer, brand and generic names, and FDA approval date here: Eli Lilly's *Prozac* (fluoxetine hydrochloride), approved by the U.S. Food and Drug Administration in 1987; Pfizer's *Zoloft* (sertraline hydrochloride), approved in 1991; Glaxo-SmithKline's *Paxil* (paroxetine hydrochloride), approved in 1992; Wyeth Pharmaceutical's *Effexor* (venlafaxine hydrochloride), approved in 1993; Forest Labs' *Celexa* (citalopram hydrobromide), approved in 1998; Forest Labs' *Lexapro* (escitalopram oxalate), approved in 2002; and Eli Lilly's *Cymbalta* (duloxetine hydrochloride), approved in 2004.

5. See, for example, Peter Conrad, *The Medicalization of Society: On the Transformation of Human Conditions into Treatable Disorders* (Baltimore: Johns Hopkins University Press, 2007).

6. David Healey, "Good Science or Good Business?" in *Prozac as a Way of Life*, ed. Carl Elliott and Tod Chambers (Chapel Hill: University of North Carolina Press, 2004), 77.

7. Allan V. Horwitz, Jerome C. Wakefield, and Robert L. Spitzer, *The Loss of Sadness: How Psychiatry Transformed Normal Sorrow into Depressive Disorder* (New York: Oxford University Press, 2007), 4.

8. For example, see David Healy, *Let Them Eat Prozac* (New York: NYU Press, 2004); Ray Moynihan and Alan Cassels, *Selling Sickness* (New York: Nation Books, 2005); and

Peter Kramer, *Against Depression* (New York: Viking, 2005). One exception is Jonathan Metzl's *Prozac on the Couch* (Durham, N.C.: Duke University Press, 2003), which reads medical and psychiatric journals, popular news reports, and pharmaceutical advertisements against the cultural scripts of psychoanalysis and biological psychiatry. Even in this important work, however, Metzl's attention to texts is limited to their ability to *reflect* cultural assumptions and categories.

9. William Styron, *Darkness Visible* (New York: Random House, 1990), 37.

10. Irving Kirsch, Brett J. Deacon, Tania B. Huedo-Medina, Alan Scoboria, Thomas J. Moore, and Blair T. Johnson, "Initial Severity and Antidepressant Benefits: A Meta-Analysis of Data Submitted to the Food and Drug Administration," *PLoS Medicine* 5, no. 2 (2008). Available: http://medicine.plosjournals.org/perlserv/?request=get-document&doi=10.1371/journal.pmed.0050045&ct=1#top. Accessed: March 1, 2008.

11. CES-D threshold scores (11–29 indicate mild to moderate symptoms) were derived from Marie-Annette Brown and Jo Robinson, *When Your Body Gets the Blues* (New York: St. Martin's Press, 2002), 177; Myrna M. Weissman et al., "Assessing Depressive Symptoms in Five Psychiatric Populations: A Validation Study," *American Journal of Epidemiology* 106, no. 3 (1977): 203–213; and H. C. Schulberg et al., "Assessing Depression in Primary Medical and Psychiatric Practices," *Archives of General Psychiatry* 42, no. 12 (1985): 1164–1170.

12. Gay Eade and Julie Bradshaw, "Understanding Discourses of the Worried Well," *Australian and New Zealand Journal of Mental Health Nursing* 4 (1995): 61–69.

13. For more on ethnographic interviewing, see James P. Spradley, *The Ethnographic Interview* (Fort Worth, Tex.: Harcourt College Publishers, 1979); Elliot G. Mishler, *Research Interviewing: Context and Narrative* (Cambridge, Mass.: Harvard University Press, 1986); Ruthellen Josselson, ed., *Ethics and Process in the Narrative Study of Lives* (Thousand Oaks, Calif.: Sage, 1996).

14. See Healy, *Let Them Eat Prozac*, for a description of the counterdiscourses, including critiques of the pharmaceutical industry for withholding information.

15. As Judy Z. Segal explains, this is a common use of what classical rhetoric calls epideictic rhetoric. See her *Health and the Rhetoric of Medicine* (Carbondale: Southern Illinois University Press, 2005).

1. DEPRESSION, A RHETORICAL ILLNESS

1. See, for example, Dana Crowley Jack, *Silencing the Self* (Cambridge, Mass.: Harvard University Press, 1991); Nell Casey, *Unholy Ghost* (New York: William Morrow, 2001).

2. For a review of the "he/man" debate, see Wendy Martyna, "Beyond the 'He/Man' Approach: The Case for Nonsexist Language," *Signs* 5, no. 3 (Spring 1980): 482–493. Critics of the feminist movement suggested that such changes were unnecessary because they were simply cosmetic, or were forms of "political correctness" in its pejorative meaning. See Deborah Cameron, *Verbal Hygiene* (New York: Routledge, 1995), especially chapter 4, for a nuanced reading of the political correctness movement.

3. Laura D. Hirschbein, "Science, Gender, and the Emergence of Depression in American Psychiatry, 1952–1980," *Journal of the History of Medicine and Allied Sciences* 61, no. 2 (2006): 202.

4. For a more complete articulation of the argument that diseases have been *created*, see Ray Moynihan and Alan Cassels, *Selling Sickness* (New York: Nation Books, 2005);

David Healy, *Let Them Eat Prozac* (New York: NYU Press, 2004); Allan V. Horwitz, Jerome C. Wakefield, and Robert L. Spitzer, *The Loss of Sadness: How Psychiatry Transformed Normal Sorrow into Depressive Disorder* (New York: Oxford University Press, 2007).

5. Andrew Lakoff, *Pharmaceutical Reason: Knowledge and Value in Global Psychiatry* (Cambridge: Cambridge University Press, 2005), 7.

6. Michel Foucault, *Madness and Civilization: A History of Insanity in the Age of Reason*, trans. Richard Howard (New York: Vintage Books, 1988).

7. Lilie Chouliaraki and Norman Fairclough, *Discourse in Late Modernity: Rethinking Critical Discourse Analysis* (Edinburgh: Edinburgh University Press, 1999), 4.

8. Ibid., 6.

9. Lawrence Rubin, "Psychotropia: Medicine, Media, and the Virtual Asylum," *Journal of Popular Culture* 39, no. 2 (2006): 262.

10. Ibid. See also David Healy, *The Antidepressant Era* (Cambridge, Mass.: Harvard University Press, 1997); Charles Barber, *Comfortably Numb: How Psychiatry Is Medicating a Nation* (New York: Pantheon Books, 2008); Ray Moynihan and Alan Cassels, *Selling Sickness* (New York: Nation Books, 2005).

11. John M. Grahol, "An Introduction to Depression," *PsychCentral*, Dec. 6, 2006. Available: <http://www.psychcentral.com/disorders/depression/>. Accessed: June 20, 2007.

12. Carl Elliott and Todd Chambers, eds., *Prozac as a Way of Life* (Durham: University of North Carolina Press, 2004), 4.

13. Lauren Slater, *Prozac Diary* (New York: Penguin Books, 1998); Persimmon Blackbridge, *Prozac Highway* (New York: Marion Boyars, 1997); Peter Kramer, *Listening to Prozac* (New York: Penguin Books, 1993); Jonathan Metzl, *Prozac on the Couch* (Durham, N.C.: Duke University Press, 2003); Healy, *Let Them Eat Prozac*; Elliott and Chambers, eds., *Prozac as a Way of Life*; Joseph Glenmullen, *Prozac Backlash* (New York: Touchstone, 2000).

14. Elizabeth Wurtzel, *Prozac Nation: A Memoir* (Boston/New York: Houghton Mifflin, 1994), 302–303.

15. Martha Manning, *Undercurrents: A Life beneath the Surface* (San Francisco: Harper, 1995), 165.

16. Carl Elliot, *Better than Well: American Medicine Meets the American Dream* (New York: W. W. Norton, 2003).

17. Lewis Wolpert, *Malignant Sadness: The Anatomy of Depression* (New York: Free Press, 1999), 176.

18. The current version of the *DSM*, including descriptive rather than etiological (psychodynamic) terminology, is, according to Kirk and Kutchins, an invention of the third edition (1980), which signaled the American Psychiatric Association's turn toward research and biological psychiatry. For more on the development of the *DSM*, see Stuart A. Kirk and Herb Kutchins, *The Selling of DSM: The Rhetoric of Science in Psychiatry* (New York: Aldine de Gruyter, 1992); Herb Kutchins and Stuart A. Kirk, *Making Us Crazy DSM: The Psychiatric Bible and the Creation of Mental Disorders* (New York: Free Press, 1997); and Shorter, *A History of Psychiatry* (New York: John Wiley and Sons, 1997), esp. 298–305.

19. Robert L. Spitzer, "Foreword," in Horwitz et al. *The Loss of Sadness*, vii.

20. Ibid.

21. Gerald L. Klerman, "The Contemporary American Scene," in *Sources and Traditions of Classification in Psychiatry*, ed. Norman Sartorius et al. (Toronto: Hogrefe and Huber, 1990), 94.

22. American Psychiatric Association, *Diagnostic and Statistical Manual: Mental Disorders* (DSM-I) (Washington, D.C.: American Psychiatric Association, 1952), v.

23. John Frederick Reynolds, David C. Mair, and Pamela C. Fisher, *Writing and Reading Mental Health Records: Issues and Analysis* (Newbury Park, Calif.: Sage Publications, 1992), 67.

24. American Psychiatric Association, *DSM-I*, 46.

25. American Psychiatric Association, *Diagnostic and Statistical Manual of Mental Disorders: Third Ed.* (DSM-III) (Washington, D.C.: American Psychiatric Association, 1980), 2.

26. Ibid., 1.

27. Ibid., 12.

28. American Psychiatric Association, *Diagnostic and Statistical Manual of Mental Disorders: Third Ed. Rev.* (DSM-III-R) (Washington, D.C.: American Psychiatric Association, 1987), xxvi.

29. American Psychiatric Association, *Diagnostic and Statistical Manual of Mental Disorders: Fourth Ed. Text Rev.* (DSM-IV-TR) (Washington, D.C.: American Psychiatric Association, 2000), 8.

30. Ibid., xxiii.

31. Ibid., xxxii.

32. Ibid., xxxiii.

33. Ibid., 349.

34. David Karp, *Speaking of Sadness* (New York: Oxford University Press, 1996), 14.

35. Jennifer Radden, ed., *The Nature of Melancholy: From Aristotle to Kristeva* (New York: Oxford University Press, 2000), 44.

36. Stanley Jackson, *Melancholia and Depression: From Hippocratic Times to Modern Times* (New Haven: Yale University Press, 1986), 404.

37. Karp, *Speaking of Sadness*, 28.

38. National Institute of Mental Health, *Depression: What Every Woman Should Know* (Bethesda, Md.: National Institutes of Health, U.S. Department of Health and Human Services, 2006) (NIH Publication No. 05–4779).

39. Kramer, *Listening to Prozac*, 18.

40. Ibid., 19.

41. Ibid., xvi.

42. John P. Hewitt, Michael R. Fraser, and LeslieBeth Berger, "Is It Me or Is It Prozac? Antidepressants and the Construction of the Self," in *Pathology and the Postmodern*, ed. Dwight Fee (Thousand Oaks, Calif.: Sage, 2000), 179.

43. Peter Kramer, *Against Depression* (New York: Viking, 2005), 4.

44. Justine Coupland and Richard Gwyn, eds., *Discourse, the Body, and Identity* (New York: Palgrave, 2003), 4.

45. Kenneth J. Gergen, *The Saturated Self: Dilemma of Identity in Contemporary Life* (New York: Basic Books, 1991), 14–15.

46. For an analysis and history of advice directed at women, see Barbara Ehrenreich and Deirdre English, *For Her Own Good: 150 Years of the Experts' Advice to Women* (1978; New York: Anchor Books, 1989).

47. Jack, *Silencing the Self*, 27 (emphasis added).

48. World Health Organization, "Gender" (2008). Available: http://www.who.int/topics/gender/en/. Accessed: March 1, 2008.

49. Ibid.

50. See, for example, Michael C. Miller, "Stop Pretending Nothing's Wrong," *Newsweek* 141, no. 24 (June 16, 2003): 71.

51. While most contemporary texts are carefully neutral on matters of class and race, the underlying assumptions—that one has time and insurance coverage (or disposable income) to allow for talk therapy or pharmaceutical intervention, for example—clearly target a middle-class, often white, individual.

52. Meri Nana-Ama Danquah, *Willow Weep for Me* (New York: One World/Ballantine, 1999), 21.

53. John Langone, "Quiet Demons in Black Life," *New York Times*, 7 December 2003, F7.

54. The 1990 APA Taskforce on Women and Depression is a good indicator of the attention paid specifically to women's depression. See Ellen McGrath and Gwendolyn Puryear Keita, eds., *Women and Depression: Risk Factors and Treatment Issues* (Washington, D.C.: American Psychological Association, 1990).

55. National Institute of Mental Health, *Women Hold Up Half the Sky* (2000). Available: http://www.nimh.nih.gov/publicat/womensoms.cfm.

56. World Health Organization, *The Global Burden of Disease* (2000). Available: http://ww.who.int/msa/mnh/ems/dalys/intro.htm.

57. See also Radden, ed., *Nature of Melancholy*, 39.

58. Susan Nolen-Hoeksema, *Sex Differences in Depression* (Stanford, Calif.: Stanford University Press, 1993), 6.

59. Ibid., 43.

60. See, for example, Phyllis Chesler, *Women and Madness* (New York: Avon Books, 1972).

61. McGrath's book is less interested in social influences on depression than Chesler's—aside from suggesting that societal pressures on women (to be young, to be thin, to be beautiful) exist. McGrath's discussion of "Healthy Depression" focuses on the ways that individuals should learn to cope with these expectations. *When Feeling Bad Is Good* (New York: Henry Holt, 1992) is an interesting artifact both for the ways that it tries to demarcate the boundaries of illness and for the ways it reasserts appropriate subjectivities.

62. Kramer, *Against Depression,* 255.

63. While statistics indicate that suicide is more often successful in men, more women attempt it each year, so, while this example might reasonably be read as addressing both women and men, it cannot be read as establishing "gender equity."

64. Ibid., 257.

65. A similar elision of fathers is present in Andrew Solomon's *Noonday Demon: An Atlas of Depression* (New York: Sailres, 2001). He writes: "To improve the mental health of children, it is sometimes more important to treat the *mother* than to treat the children directly; to try to change negative *familial patterns* to incorporate flexibility,

hardiness, cohesion, and problem-solving ability. . . . Children of depressed *mothers* have more difficulties in the world than do children of schizophrenic *mothers*: depression has a singularly immediate effect on the basic mechanisms of *parenting*" (181, emphasis added). Additional examples can be found in Linda M. Blum and Nena F. Stracuzzi, "Gender in the Prozac Nation: Popular Discourse and Productive Femininity," *Gender and Society* 18, no. 3 (June 2004): 269–286.

66. National Institute of Mental Health, *Depression* (Bethesda, Md.: National Institutes of Health, U.S. Department Health and Human Services, 2000) (NIH Publication No. 00–3561).

67. NIMH, *Depression: What Every Woman Should Know*, np.

2. ARTICULATE DEPRESSION

1. *Oxford English Dictionary*, 2nd online edition.

2. United States Government Accountability Office, *Prescription Drugs: Improvements Needed in FDA's Oversight of Direct-to-Consumer Advertising* (Publication No. GAO-07–54) (Washington, D.C.: U.S. Government Accountability Office), November 2006. Available: http://www.gao.gov/new.items/d0754.pdf. Accessed: March 1, 2008.

3. For an analysis of traditional medical expertise, see Howard Waitzkin, *The Politics of Medical Encounters: How Patients and Doctors Deal with Social Problems* (New Haven: Yale University Press, 1993); for additional discussion on the discourses of medicine, see Eliot G. Mishler, *The Discourse of Medicine: Dialectics of Medical Interviews* (Norwood, N.J.: Ablex, 1984).

4. It is not the purpose of this text to debate the clinical findings supporting the use of antidepressant drug therapies. For more detailed analyses of these findings, see, for example, David Healy, *Let Them Eat Prozac* (New York: NYU Press, 2004); Jonathan Metzl, *Prozac on the Couch* (Durham, N.C.: Duke University Press, 2003); Joseph Glenullen, *Prozac Backlash* (New York: Touchstone, 2000); Ray Moynihan and Alan Cassels, *Selling Sickness* (New York: Nation Books, 2005). I concede from the outset that these drugs do a lot of good for a lot of people. My concern, however, is with the rhetoric that surrounds the drugs and their uses, which fundamentally shapes our notions of health and illness. Individuals come to understand their experiences as constituting *depression* and as requiring medication through the language that surrounds them.

5. The collection *Prozac as a Way of Life* (ed. Carl Eliot and Todd Chambers [Chapel Hill: University of North Carolina Press, 2004]) draws together a variety of scholars to examine the effects of Prozac on social life. Some argue that it serves as an "enhancement technology" or a tool for self-creation rather than a necessary medical intervention. Indeed, some of the authors in that collection take Prozac and its marketing to be an important development on the road to drugs such as Viagra. One of the most vocal supporters of Prozac as a necessary medical intervention has been Peter Kramer, *Listening to Prozac* (New York: Penguin Books, 1993), and *Against Depression* (New York: Viking, 2005).

6. For a history of psychiatry, an excellent and concise overview is Edward Shorter, *A History of Psychiatry*, (New York: John Wiley and Sons, 1997). In addition, Jonathan Metzl reviews the twentieth-century shift toward biological psychiatry in *Prozac on the Couch*, especially chapter 2.

7. This point is made and elaborated on in two important texts: broadly, Kirk and Kutchins trace the development of the *DSM-III* and the attention it pays to specific kinds of psychiatry (*The Selling of DSM* [New York: Aldine de Gruyter, 1992]). In addition, Reyolds et al. analyze the impact of the *DSM* in clinical practice, and argue that its force as a controlling genre makes it a site worthy of close linguistic and rhetorical attention (*Writing and Reading Mental Health Records* [Newbury Park, Calif.: Sage Publications, 1992]).

8. Shorter, *A History of Psychiatry*, 288.

9. A variety of excellent histories of depression provide context for my arguments here, but none addresses the language of depression specifically. In *Prozac on the Couch*, Metzl argues that contemporary biological psychiatry reinscribes psychoanalytic categories; Jennifer Radden, *The Nature of Melancholy* (New York: Oxford University Press, 2000), provides primary sources on depression beginning with Aristotle; Stanley Jackson, *Melancholia and Depression: From Hippocratic Times to Modern Times* (New Haven: Yale University Press, 1986), remains the most cited comprehensive source for a history of depression; Christopher M. Calahan and German E. Berrios, *Reinventing Depression: A History of the Treatment of Depression in Primary Care, 1940–2004* (New York: Oxford University Press, 2004), traces the evolution of depression within primary care settings in the twentieth century.

10. World Health Organization, "Depression" (2008). Available: http://www.who.int/mental_health/management/depression/definition/en/ Accessed: March 1, 2008.

11. Andrew Lakoff, *Pharmaceutical Reason: Knowledge and Value in Global Psychiatry* (Cambridge: Cambridge University Press, 2005), 7.

12. Kramer, *Against Depression*, 39.

13. In this sentiment, Kramer echoes (and cites) Susan Sontag's classic argument against metaphoric uses of illness. For Sontag, "the most truthful way of regarding illness—and the healthiest way of being ill—is one most purified of, most resistant to, metaphoric thinking" (Susan Sontag, *Illness as Metaphor and AIDS and Its Metaphors* [1978; New York: Anchor Books, 1990], 3).

14. Peter Kramer, *Against Depression*, 9.

15. Ibid.

16. Ibid., 3.

17. Lewis Wolpert, *Malignant Sadness: The Anatomy of Depression* (New York: Free Press, 1999), 76.

18. Nell, Casey, *Unholy Ghost* (New York: William Mocraw, 2001), 2.

19. In October 2001, this advertisement appeared in *Time*, *Newsweek*, and the *New York Times Magazine*, among other places. Glaxo-SmithKline was not the only company capitalizing on the fears engendered by the events of September 11, 2001. For example, an October 2001 advertisement transformed Pfizer's Zoloft-for-depression campaign—in which the depressed creature (a cartoon sphere) sits crying under the overhang of a cliff—into a Zoloft-for-anxiety campaign by morphing the cliff into a menacing presence, which looms over the same spherical creature, now shaking with fear. The close connection between anxiety and depression has been documented in the scientific literature as well as in the popular imagination. See, for example, Holly Hazlett-Stevens, *Women Who Worry Too Much: How to Stop Worry and Anxiety from Ruining Relationships, Work and Fun* (San Francisco: New Harbinger Publications, 2005),

for a popular self-help text; and Siegfried Kasper, Johan A. den Boer, and J. M. Ad Sitsen, eds., *Handbook of Depression and Anxiety*, 2nd ed. (New York: Marcel Dekker, 2003), for an overview of the scientific literature.

20. Chapter 3 takes up the *Diagnostic and Statistical Manual of Mental Disorders* and the various definitions, both institutional and public, that constitute depression.

21. The mental health professionals in my interview comprehend symptoms as a *relationship* between experience and affect—they are less likely to judge lived experiences categorically, as these pharmaceutical ads encourage readers to do. Nevertheless, they are not immune to the shaping of illness through such repeated images and lists of symptoms.

22. Michael S. Wilkes, Robert A. Bell, and Richard L. Kravitz, "Direct-to-Consumer Prescription Drug Advertising: Trends, Impact, and Implications," *Drug Advertising* 19, no. 2 (2000): 115.

23. Michel Foucault, *Ethics: Subjectivity and Truth*, vol. 1, ed. Paul Rabinow (New York: New Press, 1997), 225.

24. Judith Butler, *Excitable Speech: A Politics of the Performative* (New York and London: Routledge, 1997), 51 (emphasis in the original).

25. Foucault, *Ethics*, 291–292.

26. Ibid., 299.

27. See Lois McNay, *Foucault and Feminism* (Boston: Northeastern University Press, 1993); Arthur Frank, "Stories of Illness as Care of the Self: A Foucauldian Dialogue," *Health* 2, no. 3 (July 1998): 329–348.

28. Judy Z. Segal, *Health and the Rhetoric of Medicine*, (Carbondale: Southern Illinois University Press, 2005), 158.

29. Ibid., 156.

30. Emily Martin, *Bipolar Expeditions: Mania and Depression in American Culture* (Princeton, N.J.: Princeton University Press, 2007), 134.

31. Ibid., xix.

32. Ibid., 10.

33. Andrew Solomon, *The Noonday Demon: An Atlas of Depression* (New York: Scribner, 2001), 300.

34. Ibid.

35. Ibid.

36. Dorothy Smith, *Texts, Facts, and Femininity: Exploring the Relations of Ruling* (London and New York: Routledge, 1990), 192–193.

37. Foucault, *Ethics*, 325.

38. Michel Foucault, *The Care of the Self: The History of Sexuality*, vol. 3, trans. Robert Hurley (New York: Vintage Books, 1986), 57.

39. Ibid., 51.

40. Michel deCerteau, *The Practice of Everyday Life*, trans. Steven Rendall (Berkeley: University of California Press, 1984), 37.

41. Ibid.

42. Ibid., 35–36.

43. Ibid., 36 (original emphasis).

44. Going to this Web site leads readers to a question: "How are depression and anxiety disorders treated?" The answer is medication, not psychotherapy or any variety of dialogic care: "Many kinds of medicines help treat these disorders."

45. The semantic gender of *guy* is, perhaps, not always straightforwardly male in contemporary usage. The colloquial phrase "you guys" can refer, in some speakers' lexicon, to a group of all women. However, in this case, Paige's other statements in the interview give me confidence that she is, indeed, assigning a male gender to the power in the advertisement.

3. STRATEGIC IMPRECISION AND THE SELF-DOCTORING DRIVE

1. William H. Gass, "Introduction" *Anatomy of Melancholy* (New York: New York Review of Books, 2001), ix.

2. Juliana Schiesari, *The Gendering of Melancholia: Feminism, Psychoanalysis, and the Symbolics of Loss in Renaissance Literature* (Ithaca, N.Y.: Cornell University Press, 1992), argues for the feminization of depression in Early Modern texts and culture.

3. National Institute of Mental Health, *Depression: What Every Woman Should Know* (Bethesda, Md: National Institutes of Health, U.S. Department Health and Human Services, 2006) (NIH Publication No. 05–4779).

4. Ibid.

5. William Styron, *Darkness Visible,* (New York: Random House, 1990), 36.

6. Ibid 36–37.

7. Lewis Wolpert, *Malignant Sadness: The Anatomy of Depression* (New York: Free Press, 1999), xii.

8. See, for example, Arthur Frank, *The Wounded Storyteller: Body, Illness, and Ethics* (Chicago: University of Chicago Press, 1995).

9. Meri Nana-Ama Danquah, *Willow Weep for Me* (New York: One World/Ballantine, 1999), 86.

10. Ibid.

11. Elizabeth Wurtzel, *Prozac Nation: A Memoir* (Boston/New York: Houghton Miffin, 1994), 59–60.

12. Ibid., 60.

13. Martha Manning, *Undercurrents: A Life Beneath the Surface* (San Francisco: Harper, 1999), 75.

14. In Myrna Weissman and Eugene Paykel's *The Depressed Woman: A Study of Social Relationships* (Chicago: University of Chicago Press, 1974), the authors describe the term *depression* as having "at least three or four meanings . . . a mood, a symptom, a syndrome, and, some would maintain, a disease or group of diseases" (1). They wish to discuss depression as a *syndrome* (*disease* is eschewed as "more controversial"), and they define *syndrome* as "borrowed from medicine and refer[ring] to a cluster of symptoms and functional disturbances that usually have a common mechanism but a variety of causes" (4). The term *syndrome* appears eighteen times in my discourse sample, but only three in reference to depression. Other references include "empty nest syndrome" (Anemona Hartocollis, "Early Pangs of Empty Nest Syndrome When the Children Leave Home for College," *New York Times* [September 4, 2005]: 34); "mean-girl syndrome" ("Action Strategies," *Blues Buster* 2, no. 6 [June 2002]: 1–2); and

"premenstrual syndrome" (e.g., "Dietary Supplement Found to Be Contaminated," *New York Times* [September 1, 1998]). One reference is masculine inflected: "John Wayne syndrome" (Peg Tyre, "Battling the Effects of War (Cover Story)," *Newsweek* 144, no. 23 [December 6, 2004]: 68–70.). Others are at least ostensibly gender neutral: "chronic fatigue syndrome" (Pat Wingert et al., "Young and Depressed," *Newsweek* 140, no. 15 [October 7, 2002]: 52); "carpal tunnel syndrome" (Sarah Kershaw, "Hooked on the Web: Help Is on the Way," *New York Times* [December 2005]: 1.). Because there are so few references to depression as a syndrome, I have not included it in my analysis. Nevertheless, the stereotypical gender collocations provide further evidence medical attention is directed at women's emotionality (as well as men's physicality).

15. Arthur Kleinman, *The Illness Narratives: Suffering, Healing and the Human Condition* (New York: Basic Books, 1988), 4.

16. Ibid., 5–6.

17. Christopher Boorse, "On the Distinction between Disease and Illness," *Philosophy and Public Affairs* 5, no. 1 (Autumn 1975): 56.

18. These definitions come from the *Oxford English Dictionary*, online 2nd edition (1989).

19. Wolpert, *Malignant Sadness*, 12.

20. Peter Kramer *Against Depression*, (New York: Viking, 2005), xiii.

21. Tracy Thompson, *The Beast: A Journey through Depression* (New York: Plume, 1996), 189.

22. NIMH, *Depression*, np.

23. Yahlin Chang, "Women Behaving Badly," *Newsweek* 131, no. 14 (April 6, 1998): 66.

24. "Blacks and the Blues," *Blues Buster* 3, no. 7 (September 2003): 1, 4–5.

25. Debra Rosenberg and Matthew Cooper. "Tipper Steps Out (Cover Story)," *Newsweek* 133, no. 21 (May 24, 1999): 48.

26. Michael D. Yapko, "Who Gets Depressed?" *Blues Buster* 2, no. 7 (July/August 2002): 8.

27. Danquah, *Willow Weep for Me*, 58.

28. Manning, *Undercurrents*, 70.

29. Ibid., 154.

30. Susan H. Greenberg et al., "The Baby Blues and Beyond," *Newsweek* 138, no. 1 (July 2, 2001): 26.

31. William Frosch, "Introduction," in *Handbook of Depression and Anxiety*, 2nd ed., ed. Siegfried Kasper, Johan A. den Boer, and J. M. Ad Sitsen (New York: Marcel Dekker, Inc., 2003), iii.

32. Danquah, *Willow Weep for Me*, 18.

33. Genre theorist Anne Freadman sums up the purpose of not-statements in distinguishing between genres: "Starting from the class of all texts, or discourse, the not-statement is the first move establishing a generic classification. . . . [it] gives this kind of place among other places." "Anyone for Tennis?" in *Genre and the New Rhetoric*, ed. Aviva Freedman and Peter Medway (London: Taylor and Francis, 1994), 51–52.

34. Wolpert, *Malignant Sadness*, 46.

35. "101 Facts about Depression," *Blues Buster*/4, no. 4 (May 2004), 1, 4–7.

36. Solomon, *The Noonday Demon*, 398.

37. In addition, his use of pregnancy as the categorical analogy—even as he denies depression's similarity to it—is another indication of the gendering of the illness:

women's bodies, particularly their reproductive and maternal bodies, recur throughout the discourse as objects available for interpretation, analysis, and surveillance.

38. Yapko, "Who Gets Depressed?" *Blues Buster.*

39. "Understanding Depression," *Newsweek* November 1998.

40. NIMH, *Men and Depression*, March 2003, np.

41. Ellen McGrath, "Action Strategies," *Blues Buster* 3, no. 2 (March 2003): 2.

42. "Action Strategies," *Blues Buster* 3, no. 10 (December 2003): 1–2.

43. "Blacks and the Blues," *Blues Buster.*

44. NIMH, *Depression*, np.

45. Jeffrey Smith suggests that "it's at least curious, possibly even indicative, that the word we've substituted for 'melancholia' in this century has also become synonymous with our term for a drastic economic downturn." *Where the Roots Reach for Water: A Personal and Natural History of Melancholia* (New York: New Point Press, 1999), 110.

46. NIMH, *Depression*, np.

47. McGrath, "Action Strategies," *Blues Buster* (March 2003).

48. Greenberg et al., "The Baby Blues and Beyond," 26, emphasis added.

49. Carolyn R. Miller, "Presumptions of Expertise: The Role of *Ethos* in Risk Analysis," *Configurations* 11 (2003): 166.

50. Ibid.

51. Ibid., 201.

52. Ulrich Beck, "From Industrial Society to the Risk Society: Questions of Survival, Social Structure and Ecological Enlightenment," *Theory, Culture and Society* 9 (1992): 119.

53. Ibid., 100.

54. Ibid., 119.

55. Wolpert, *Malignant Sadness*, 45.

56. Ibid., 184.

57. Linda M. Blum and Nena F. Stracuzzi, "Gender in the Prozac Nation: Popular Discourse and Productive Femininity," *Gender and Society* 18, no. 3 (June 2004): 271.

58. Michael C. Miller, "Stop Pretending Nothing's Wrong," *Newsweek* 141, no. 24 (June 16, 2003): 71.

59. Claudia H. Deutsch, "At Lunch with: Rabbi Benjamin Blech; Making a Fortune, Losing It and Moving On," *New York Times*, December 7, 2003, 8.

60. NIMH, *Depression*, np.

61. Michael C. Miller, "Stop Pretending Nothing's Wrong," *Newsweek* 141, no. 24 (June 16, 2003), 71.

62. Ibid.

63. Ibid.

64. Susan Nolen-Hoeksema, *Sex Differences in Depression* (Stanford Calif.: Stanford University Press, 1993), 6.

65. Wurtzel, *Prozac Nation*, 84.

66. Manning, *Undercurrents*, 169.

4. ISOLATING WORDS

1. See, for example, Raymond Klibansky, Erwin Panofsky, and Fritz Saxl, *Saturn and Melancholy: Studies in the History of Natural Philosophy, Religion, and Art* (New York: Basic Books, 1964).

2. Stanley Jackson, *Melancholia and Depression: From Hippocratic Times to Modern Times* (New Haven: Yale University Press, 1986), 396.

3. Ibid.

4. There are interesting parallels between these notions of color and recent developments in brain imagery. See, for example, Joseph Dumit, *Picturing Personhood: Brain Scans and Biomedical Identity* (Princeton, N.J.: Princeton University Press, 2003).

5. See, in particular, Meri Nana-Ama Danquah, *Willow Weep for Me* (New York: One World/Ballantine), 1999.

6. Jackson, *Melancholia and Depression*, 397.

7. George Lakoff and Mark Johnson, *Metaphors We Live By* (Chicago: University of Chicago Press, 1980).

8. Emily Martin, "The Egg and the Sperm: How Science Has Constructed a Romance Based on Stereotypical Male-Female Roles," *Signs* 16.3 (Spring 1991): 485–501.

9. Barbara Tomlinson, "Phallic Fables and Spermatic Romance: Disciplinary Crossing and Textual Ridicule," *Configurations* 3, no. 2 (1995): 105–134. Tomlinson focuses on the rhetorical usefulness of "textual ridicule" in critique of scientific knowledge. Emily Martin, *The Woman in the Body: A Cultural Analysis of Reproduction* (Boston: Beacon Press, 2001), provides a more detailed analysis.

10. Andrew Solomon, *The Noonday Demon: An Atlas of Depression* (New York: Scribner, 2001), 16.

11. "Crisis on Campus" *Blues Buster* 2, no. 5 (May 2002): 1, 4–5.

12. Ibid.

13. "Love and Depression," *Blues Buster* 2, no. 11 (December 2002): 1, 4–5.

14. James Dao, "The 2000 Campaign: The Family; Mrs. Gore Takes Turn on Stump," *New York Times*, June 1, 2000, 26.

15. Debra Rosenberg, "'My Ambivalence Is Pretty Normal,'" *Newsweek* 133, no. 21 (May 24, 1999): 51.

16. Lauren Slater, *Prozac Diary* (New York: Penguin Books, 1998), 10.

17. Joseph Glenmullen's *Prozac Backlash* (New York: Touchstone, 2000) documents additional side effects and results from long-term SSRI use. Slater's discussion of the treatment of sexual dysfunction as a "side effect" (and a not significant one at that) of SSRI use further argues that the *self* is divorced from its sexuality in this discourse.

18. Martha Manning, *Undercurrents: A life Beneath the Surface* (San Francisco: Harper, 1995), 196.

19. William Styron, *Darkness Visible* (New York: Random House, 1990), 79.

20. Jeffery Smith, *Where Roots Reach for Water A Personal and Natural History of Melancholia* (New York: New Point Press, 1999), 5.

21. Tracy Thompson, *The Beast: A Journey through Depression* (New York: Plume, 1996), 4.

22. Solomon, *The Noonday Demon*, 39.

23. Ibid, 15–16.

24. Michael D. Yapko, "Five Years Old and Already Blue," *Blues Buster* 4, no. 1 (January/February 2004): 8.

25. Styron, *Darkness Visible*, 32.

26. Slater, *Prozac Diary*, 11, 4.

27. Ibid., 127.

28. Joshua W. Shenk, "A Melancholy of Mine Own"; Nell Casey, ed., *Unholy Ghost: Writers on Depression* (New York: William Morrow, 2001), 247.

29. Jeffrey P. Lacasse and Jonathan Leo, "Serotonin and Depression," *PLoS Medicine* 2, no. 12 (2005). Available: http://medicine.plosjournals.org/perlserv/?request=get-document&doi=10.1371/journal.pmed.0020392. Accessed: March 1, 2008.

30. M. Sara Rosenthal, *Women and Depression* (Los Angeles: Lowell House, 2000), 157–158.

31. Thompson, *The Beast*, 253.

32. "Nourishing Your Brain." *Newsweek* 137, no. 17 (April 23, 2001): 60.

33. John Schilb, "Autobiography after Prozac," in *Rhetorical Bodies*, ed. Jack Selzer and Sharon Crowley (Madison: University of Wisconsin Press, 1999), 207.

34. Jennifer Radden, "Is This Dame Melancholy? Equating Today's Depression and Past Melancholia," *Philosophy Psychiatry and Psychology (PPP)* 10.1 (March 2003): 37–52.

35. David Karp, *Speaking of Sadness* (New York: Oxford University Press, 1996), 79.

36. Danquah, *Willow Weep for Me*, 257–258.

37. Slater, *Prozac Diary*, 24.

38. An alternative reading of these metaphors of journey is suggested by the artistic and philosophical tradition of visualizing the insane as in transit, e.g., aboard a "ship of fools." The history of containment and travel for mentally ill individuals is echoed in the narrative progression of genres like the memoir. Further, considering this cultural history, it is possible to read the women's use of journey metaphors as participating in a larger cultural narrative/memory that seeks to keep mental illness in transit (and therefore never arriving home). See Sander L. Gilman, *Disease and Representation: Images of Illness from Madness to AIDS* (Ithaca, N.Y.: Cornell University Press, 1988), for more on the history of visualizations of illness.

39. Susan Sontag, *Illness as Metaphor* (New York: Farrar, Straus and Giroux, 1978).

40. Manning, *Undercurrents*, 70.

41. Smith, *Where the Roots Reach for Water*, 60–61.

42. Michael D. Yapko, "How to Handle Difficult People," *Blues Buster* 3, no. 9 (November 2003): 8.

43. "Hearts and Minds," *Blues Buster* 3, no. 1 (January/February 2003): 1, 6–7.

44. Manning, *Undercurrents*, 186.

45. NIMH, *Men and Depression*, np.

46. Ellen McGrath, "Action Strategies," *Blues Buster* 2, no. 10 (November 2002): 1–2.

47. Pat Wingert et al., "Young and Depressed," *Newsweek* 140, no. 15 (October 7, 2002): 52.

48. Malcolm Jones Jr. and Brad Stone, "The Death of a Native Son," *Newsweek* 129, no. 17 (April 28, 1997): 82.

49. Styron, *Darkness Visible*, 40.

50. Jones, "The Death of a Native Son," *Newsweek* 129, no. 17 (April 28, 1997), 82.

51. David Gates, "Invitation to the Blues," *Newsweek* 137, no. 24 (June 11, 2001): 56.

52. Thompson, *The Beast*, 13.

53. Solomon, *The Noonday Demon*, 17.

54. Manning, *Undercurrents*, 183.

55. Frank Bruni, "Public Lives: Tipper Gore Keeps Cautious Watch at Door She Opened," *New York Times*, June 7, 1999, 16.

56. Claude Elwood Shannon, *The Mathematical Theory of Communication* (Urbana: University of Illinois Press, 1949).

57. Faye Zucker, *Depression* (New York: Franklin Watts, 2003).

58. Geoffrey Cowley and Anne Underwood, "What Is SAMe?" *Newsweek* 134, no. 1 (July 5, 1999): 46, emphasis added.

59. Erica Goode, "Power of Positive Thinking May Have a Health Benefit, Study Says," *New York Times*, September 2, 2003, 5, emphasis added.

60. Cowley and Underwood, "What Is SAMe?" 46.

61. Ellen McGrath, "Action Strategies," *Blues Buster* 2, no. 3 (March 2002): 1–2.

62. "Brain's Big Two-Fer," *Blues Buster* 3, no. 8 (October 2003): 1, 4–5.

63. Manning, *Undercurrents*, 64.

64. Solomon, *The Noonday Demon*, 129.

65. Ibid., 30.

66. Slater, *Prozac Diary*, 78.

5. TELLING STORIES OF DEPRESSION

1. Food and Drug Administration, "FDA Launches a Multi-Pronged Strategy to Strengthen Safeguards for Children Treated with Antidepressant Medications" (October 15, 2004). Available online: http://www.fda.gov/bbs/topics/news/2004/new01124.html.

2. Pfizer is not the only antidepressant manufacturer to adopt more social images in its advertising campaigns. The Cymbalta (Eli Lilly's antidepressant approved by the FDA in 2004) advertisement includes a series of vignettes accompanying each statement about depression ("Who does depression hurt?"). The Effexor advertisements of the 1990s could be read as precursors to these storylines: they included images accompanying first-person statements that implied a narrative of cure ("I got my mommy back . . . "), although they did not define the identity and social role of the cured individual ("mommy") as clearly as the 2005 Zoloft advertisement does via its complete narrative.

3. William Styron, *Darkness Visible* (New York: Random House, 1990), 3.

4. Ibid.

5. Ibid.

6. Abigail Cheever, "Prozac Americans: Depression, Identity, and Selfhood," *Twentieth Century Literature* 46.3 (Autumn, 2000): 346–368. The motif of discovery here recalls the geographical metaphors. Indeed, stories often depend on such metaphors, and, as my analysis in chapter 4 suggested, metaphors achieve much of their power from their implied narrative trajectories.

7. Andrew Solomon, *The Noonday Demon: An Atlas of Depression* (New York: Scribner, 2001), 11–12.

8. Meri Nana-Ama Danquah, *Willow Weep for Me* (New York: One World/Ballantine, 1999), 234–235.

9. Solomon, *The Noonday Demon*, 13.

10. Mary Anne Hughes, "Malignant Sadness (Book Review)," *Library Journal* 125, no. 4 (2000): III.

11. See, for example, Arthur Frank, *The Wounded Storyteller: Body, Illness, and Ethics* (Chicago: University of Chicago Press, 1995); Rita Charon, *Narrative Medicine: Honoring the Stories of Illness* (New York: Oxford University Press, 2006); Arthur Kleinman, *The Illness Narratives: Suffering, Healing and the Human Condition* (New York: Basic Books, 1988).

12. Irving Kirsch, Brett J. Deacon, Tania B. Huedo-Medina, Alan Scoboria, Thomas J. Moore, and Blair T. Johnson, "Initial Severity and Antidepressant Benefits: A Meta-Analysis of Data Submitted to the Food and Drug Administration," *PLOS Medicine* 5, no. 2 (2008).

13. Sharon Begley, "Depressing News on Antidepressants," *Newsweek*, Blog, February 25, 2008.

14. Judy Segal, "What Is a Story of Breast Cancer?" Proceedings of the 4th International Conference on Genre Studies, Tubarão, Brazil, August 2007, 160–161.

15. Arthur Frank, *At the Will of the Body* (Boston, Mass.: Houghton Mifflin: 2002), 124.

16. Ibid.

17. Talcott Parsons's description of the "sick role" provides a model for the responsibilities attendant upon the relief from social obligations (e.g., going to work) that falling ill allows. Those in the sick role must place themselves in the care of medical institutions, and they must *want* to get well. This model, as Simon Williams describes it, views the sick role as "a socially prescribed mechanism for channeling and controlling" the deviance of illness (*The Social System* [London: Routledge and Kegan Paul, 1951], 123). Williams's sympathetic rereading of Parsons provides additional insight into the value of the "sick role" in the discursive late-modern environment.

18. Ibid., 128.

19. See, for example, Robyn Fivush and Janine P. Buckner, "Gender, Sadness, and Depression: The Development of Emotional Focus through Gendered Discourse," in *Gender and Emotion: Social Psychological Perspectives*, ed. Agneta H. Fischer (Cambridge: Cambridge University Press, 2000), 232–253.

20. Frank, *The Wounded Storyteller*.

21. For more on this vocabulary, see Fivush and Buckner, "Gender, Sadness, and Depression," 223.

22. Jeffrey Smith, *Where Roots Reach for Water: A Personal and Natural History of Melancholia* (New York: New Point Press, 1999), 243.

23. Ibid., 242.

24. Ibid., 244.

25. Tracy Thompson, *The Beast: A Journey though Depression* (New York: Plume, 1996), 176.

26. Ibid., 215.

27. "Suicide: A Whole New View," *Blues Buster* 3, no. 4 (May 2003): 1, 6–7.

28. Daniel McGinn and Ron Depasquale, "Taking Depression On," *Newsweek* 144, no. 8 (August 23, 2004): 59–60.

29. A fourth occurrence refers to Howard Stern and Rosanne Barr as "unfortunate" poster children for obsessive-compulsive disorder. Jolie Solomon, Claudia Kalb, et al., "Breaking the Silence," *Newsweek* 127, no. 21 (May 20, 1996): 20.

30. John Leland, "The Night without End," *Newsweek* 134, no. 15 (October 11, 1999): 71–71.

31. "Even CEOs Get the Blues," *Blues Buster* 3, no. 2 (March 2003): 1, 4–7.

32. Ibid.

33. Ibid.

34. Ibid.

35. Burguieres's story of corporate success can be usefully read against Terry Bradshaw's story of sports fame. One article prefaces Bradshaw's depression as follows: "Terry Bradshaw had a lot to feel good about during the early 1990s. As a quarterback for the Pittsburgh Steelers, he had won four Super Bowls. He gained a spot in pro football's Hall of Fame the first year he was eligible. And, when he retired from football as a player in 1984, he made the jump to the broadcast side look easy. . . . Yet the surfeit of success left Bradshaw oddly joyless" (Michael C. Miller, "Stop Pretending Nothing's Wrong," *Newsweek* 141, no. 24 [June 16, 2003]: 71).

36. Quoted in Yahlin Chang, "Women Behaving Badly," *Newsweek* 131, no. 14 (April 6, 1998): 66.

37. Ibid.

38. Ibid.

39. Ann Burns, "Forecasts: Nonfiction," *Publishers Weekly* 245.1 (1998): 53.

40. Bonnie Hoffman, "Book Reviews: Social Sciences," *Library Journal* 120.3 (1995): 172.

41. Eve Leeman, "Answering Back to Prozac," *Lancet* 353.9147 (1999): 155.

42. David Klinghoffer, "*Prozac Nation: A Memoir* (Book Review)," *National Review* 46, no. 21 (7 November 1994): 74–76.

43. Paul Chance, "Bookworms," *Psychology Today* 33, no. 1 (2000): 72.

44. W. W. Meissner, "Life on the Line," *America* 182, no. 19 (2000): 26.

45. Peter Kavanagh et al., "Critics' Choices for Christmas," *Commonweal* 128, no. 21 (2001): 21.

46. "Depression at Work," *Blues Buster* 3, no. 10 (December 2003): 1, 4–6.

47. "The Trouble with Men," *Blues Buster* 2, no. 1 (December 2001/January 2002): 1, 6–7.

48. Howard Fineman and Michael Isikoff, "Powell on the Brink," *Newsweek* 126, no. 19 (November 6, 1995): 36.

49. NIMH, *Depression: What Every Woman Should Know*, np.

50. Ibid.

51. NIMH, *Men and Depression*, np.

52. Ibid.

53. Ibid.

54. NIMH, *Depressions: What Every Woman Should Know*, np.

55. Mary Crowley, "Do Kids Need Prozac?" *Newsweek* 130, no. 16 (October 20, 1997): 73.

56. Ibid.

57. Gail Braccidiferro, "The Frustrations of Mental Health Care," *New York Times*, March 2, 2003, 1.

58. Ibid.

59. Jane E. Brody, "Personal Health; Invisible World of the Seriously Depressed Child," *New York Times*, December 2, 1997, 9.

60. Braccidiferro, "The Frustrations of Mental Health Care," 1.

61. Ibid.

62. Pat Wingert, "Young and Depressed," *Newsweek* 140, no. 15 (October 7, 2002): 52.

63. Debra Rosenberg and Matthew Cooper, "Tipper Steps Out," *Newsweek* 133, no. 21 (May 24, 1999): 48.

64. Susan H. Greenberg et al., "The Baby Blues and Beyond," *Newsweek* 138, no. 1 (July 2, 2001): 26.

65. Anemona Hartocollis, "Early Pangs of Empty Nest Syndrome When the Children Leave Home for College," *New York Times*, September 4, 2005, 34.

66. Greenberg et al., "The Baby Blues and Beyond," *Newsweek*.

67. Michael C. Miller, "Stop Pretending Nothing's Wrong," *Newsweek* 141, no. 24 (June 16, 2003): 71.

68. Mark Miller, "To Be Gay—And Mormon," *Newsweek* 135, no. 19 (May 8, 2000): 38.

69. Terry Pristin, "Two Dead in Shooting," *New York Times*, June 6, 1997, 1.

70. Emily Martin, "The Pharmaceutical Person," *BioSocieties* 1 (2006): 273.

71. The pharmaceutical habits of men do not receive the same narrative embedding as do those of women; men's antidepressant use is most often stated as a fact followed by the event of success. For example, a 78-year-old man is "prescribed Paxil and a brief course of psychotherapy [for his depression]. The depression has lifted" ("Gaps Seen in Treating Depression in Elderly," *New York Times*, September 5, 1999). In one notable exception, Tristan Logan's decision to receive testosterone replacement therapy appears within a longer narrative. The article describes Logan: "The 55-year-old, an avid weight lifter with a black belt in tae kwon do, was tired and weak. The amount of iron he was able to pump during workouts was decreasing, after steadily increasing for years. Worse, the antidepressants he takes seemed to stop working, and his mood darkened" ("High on Testosterone," *Newsweek*, September 29, 2003). Logan's masculinity—potentially threatened by low levels of testosterone—is expressively restored via descriptions of his athletic achievements. Similar to the women whose pharmaceutical personhood is established through alternative therapies, Logan "has no plans to stop" his testosterone replacement.

72. Sue Miller, "A Natural Mood Booster," *Newsweek* 129, no. 18 (May 5, 1997): 74.

73. Ibid.

74. Cowley and Underwood, "What Is SAMe?" 46.

75. Ibid.

76. Michael D. Yapko, "What Drugs Can—and Can't—Do," *Blues Buster* 2, no. 8 (September 2002): 8.

77. Ibid.

78. Michale D. Yapko, "Who Gets to Decide What," *Blues Buster* 2, no. 2 (February 2002): 8.

79. Ibid.

80. Ibid.

81. Michael D. Yapko, "How to Get Help for a Loved One," *Blues Buster* 3, no. 1 (January/February 2003): 8.

82. Ibid.

83. Ibid.

84. Ibid., emphasis added.

85. Michael D. Yapko, "When Helplessness Drives Others Crazy," *Blues Buster* 3, no. 3 (April 2003): 8.

86. Ibid.

87. Deborah Schiffrin, *Discourse Markers* (New York: Cambridge University Press, 1987), 268.

6. DIAGNOSTIC GENRES AND THE RECONFIGURING OF MEDICAL EXPERTISE

1. For a consideration of other nosologies, see Juan E. Mezzich, Yutaka Honda, and Marianne C. Kastrup, eds., *Psychiatric Diagnosis: A World Perspective* (New York: Springer-Verlag, 1994).

2. The move of the *DSM* into the public sphere can be seen in various general-interest publications. See, for example, Spiegel, "The Dictionary of Disorder," *New Yorker*, January 3, 2005); Elliot, "A New Way to Be Mad," *Atlantic Monthly*, December 2000.

3. Carolyn R. Miller, "Genre as Social Action," in *Genre and the New Rhetoric*, ed. Aviva Freedman and Peter Medway (Bristol, Penn.: Taylor and Francis, 1994), 31.

4. For example, Catherine Schryer ("The Lab vs. the Clinic: Sites of Competing Genres," in *Genre and the New Rhetoric*, 105–124), identifies competing ideologies within a veterinary school by analyzing the laboratory and clinical genres. For more on genre theory, see the foundational collections in Aviva Freedman and Peter Medway, eds., *Genre and the New Rhetoric* (London: Taylor and Francis, 1994); Wendy Bishop and Hans Ostrom, eds., *Genre and Writing: Issues, Arguments, Alternatives* (Portsmouth, N.H.: Boynton/Cook, 1997); Richard Coe, Lorelei Lingard, and Tatiana Teslenko, eds., *The Rhetoric and Ideology of Genre: Strategies for Stability and Change* (Cresskill, N.J.: Hampton Press, 2002).

5. See, for example, Charles Bazerman, "Discursively Structured Activities," *Mind, Culture, and Activity* 4.4 (1997): 296–308; and Anis Bawarshi, *Genre and the Invention of the Writer* (Logan: Utah State University Press, 2003), especially chapter 5; Anne Freadman, "Uptake," in *The Rhetoric and Ideology of Genre*, 39–53.

6. Steven Woloshin et al., "Direct-to-Consumer Advertisements for Prescription Drugs: What Are Americans Being Sold?" *The Lancet* 358 (2001): 1146.

7. Michael S.Wilkes, Robert A. Bell, and Richard L. Kravitz, "Direct-to-Consumer Prescription Drug Advertising: Trends, Impact, and Implications," *Drug Advertising* 19.2 (2000): 115.

8. Ibid.

9. See, for example, L. R. Krupka and A. M. Vener, "Gender Differences in Drug (Prescription, Non-Prescription, Alcohol and Tobacco) Advertising: Trends and Implications," *Journal of Drug Issues* 22, no. 2 (1992): 339–360. In addition, print and online advertisements for WebMD (available: http://www.webmd.com), a popular online source for health information, promote discussions with both medical professionals and also nonmedical celebrities as opportunities to talk about health issues.

10. A similar joke underlies the *Shouts and Murmurs* column by Louis Menand, "Listening to Bourbon," *New Yorker*, April 18, 1994, 108.

11. Poe is a particular favorite of *New Yorker* cartoonists, and his potential "cure" via Prozac inspires "Edgar Allan Prozac" (who dreams of white doves instead of ravens) in Drew Dernavich's November 2006 cartoon, and the "bluebird of Prozac" in Robert Mankoff's August 1993 cartoon.

12. Carol Berkenkotter, "Genre Systems at Work: DSM-IV and Rhetorical Recontextualization in Psychotherapy Paperwork," *Written Communication* 18, no. 3 (2001): 330.

13. Ibid., 330.

14. Ibid., 334.

15. Hannah Lerman, *Pigeonholing Women's Misery: A History and Critical Analysis of the Psychodiagnosis of Women in the Twentieth Century* (New York: Basic Books, 1996), 5.

16. In addition to the concerns about influences on "objective" diagnoses, feminists have focused critical energy on exploring the ways that science has been used historically to control women's minds and bodies. Jill Astbury's *Crazy for You: The Making of Women's Madness* (Oxford: Oxford University Press, 1996) offers this kind of analysis, considering diagnoses like hysteria, depression, and battered child syndrome.

17. Joan Busfield, *Men, Women and Madness: Understanding Gender and Mental Disorder* (New York: New York University Press, 1996), 94.

18. These and other quizzes are available in the "Love & Sex" subsection of the "women's community online" iVillage.com (http://www.ivillage.com). Additional, health-related quizzes are available from the "Health and Well-Being" subsection of the same site.

19. American Psychiatric Association, *Diagnostic and Statistical Manual of Mental Disorders: Fourth Ed. Text Rev. (DSM-IV-TR)* (Washington, D.C.: American Psychiatric Association, 2000), 356.

20. See, for example, Carol Berkenkotter, "Genre Systems at Work: DSM-IV and Rhetorical Recontextualization in Psychotherapy Paperwork," *Written Communication* 18, no. 3 (2001): 326–349; Carol Berkenkotter and Doris Ravotas, "New Research Strategies in Genre Analysis: Reported Speech as Recontextualization in a Psychotherapist's Notes and Initial Assessment," in *Discourse Studies in Composition*, ed. Ellen Barton and Gail Stygall (Cresskill, N.J.: Hampton Press, 2001), 229–256; Carol Berkenkotter and Doris Ravotas, "Genre as Tool in the Transmission of Practice over Time and across Professional Boundaries," *Mind, Culture, and Activity* 4, no. 4 (1997): 256–274.

21. In 1997, the U.S. Food and Drug Administration (FDA) released guidelines for direct-to-consumer advertising that significantly relaxed the regulation of such marketing efforts. See, for example, Steven Findlay, *Prescription Drugs and Mass Media Advertising* (Washington, D.C.: National Institute of Health Care Management, 2000) Available: http://www.nihcm.org/~nihcmor/pdf/DTCbrief2001.pdf. Accessed: March 10, 2008.

22. As evidence of such popular interest, consider memoirs like Elizabeth Wurtzel's *Prozac Nation* (Boston/New York: Houghton Mifflin, 1994), which became a feature film of the same name (Dir. Erik Skjoldbjærg, Miramax, 2001), and nonfiction best-sellers like Peter Kramer's *Listening to Prozac* (New York: Penguin Books, 1993).

23. See, for example, the Pfizer's "Depression Checklist," available from the Zoloft Web site: http://www.zoloft.com/zoloft/zoloft.portal?_nfpb=true&_pageLabel=depr_checklist.

24. Prozac advertisement, *Time*, February 9, 1998, 98, emphasis added.

25. Zoloft advertisement, *Newsweek*, June 25, 2001, 58.

26. The measurement tools upon which these quizzes are based were developed in 1965 (W.W.K. Zung, "A Self-Rating Depression Scale," *Archives of General Psychiatry* 12 [1965]: 63–70); 1971 (Center for Epidemiologic Studies, National Institute of Mental Health, *Center for Epidemiologic Studies Depression Scale [CES-D]* [Rockville, Md.: National Institute of Mental Health, 1971]); and 1995 (R. L. Spitzer et al., *Prime-MD: Clinical Evaluation Guide* [Pfizer, 1995]). The *DSM-IV-TR* was published in 2000. Pfizer, the manufacturer of Zoloft, supported the development of the PRIME-MD. Given the disparate publication dates of the underlying measurement tools and the uncertainties of the exact dates of the quiz versions (though the Web sites have appeared only recently), tracing an "uptake timeline" from one document to the next would be fruitless. Rather, I mean to suggest that *all* of these documents participate in the processes of discursive uptake that help reinforce the current (2008) definition of depression.

27. Further, the Prozac.com quiz directs the following: "If you are on a diet, answer statements 5 and 7 as if you were not."

28. Emily Martin, *Bipolar Expeditions: Mania and Depression in American Culture* (Princeton, N.J.: Princeton University Press, 2007), 183.

29. Arthur Kleinman, "Who We Are: Illness and Other Dangers to Everyday Moral Experience," Keynote Lecture, Case Western Reserve University, March 22, 2004.

30. The mental health professionals whom I interviewed suggested, for example, that aggression and excessive anger were sometimes linked to an underlying depressive disorder.

31. The psychiatric redefinition of *sadness* as *depression* is the subject of Allan V. Horwitz, Jerome C. Wakefield, and Robert L. Spitzer, *The Loss of Sadness: How Psychiatry Transformed Normal Sorrow into Depressive Disorder* (New York: Oxford University Press, 2007).

CONCLUSION: TOWARD A RHETORICAL CARE OF THE SELF

1. Lauren Slater, *Prozac Diary* (New York: Penguin Books, 1998), 11.

2. Ibid., 4–5.

3. Ibid., 6.

4. Ibid., 8.

5. Rita Charon, *Narrative Medicine: Honoring the Stories of Illness* (New York and Oxford: Oxford University Press, 2006), viii.

6. Ibid.

7. Ibid., vii (emphasis added).

8. Ibid., vii, 3.

9. Something like this is implied in Cheryl Mattingly, *Healing Dramas and Clinical Plots: The Narrative Structure of Experience* (New York: Cambridge University Press, 1998). Mattingly finds that patients who can construct successful narratives recover more quickly from their illnesses.

10. Charon, *Narrative Medicine*, 132.

11. Ibid., 149.

12. "Taking Depression On," *Newsweek*, August 23, 2004.

INDEX

ABOUT THE AUTHOR

KIMBERLY K. EMMONS is an associate professor of English and director of composition at Case Western Reserve University. Her work has appeared in various writing journals and medical rhetoric collections, including *Composition Studies, The Rhetoric of Healthcare,* and *Genre in a Changing World.* At Case Western Reserve, she teaches undergraduate and graduate courses in composition theory and pedagogy; the history of English; language and gender; and medical rhetoric.